ENERGY HEALING

ENERGY HEALING

— REFLECTIONS ON A JOURNEY —

MARY SZCZEPANSKI

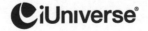

ENERGY HEALING
REFLECTIONS ON A JOURNEY

Illustrations and credits
Figure 1 Marcia Mulloy (and help with all graphics preparation)
Figure 2 Layout Patti Restaino, figure by Marcia Mulloy
Figure 3 Zara Sykes
Figure 4 Zara Sykes
Figure 5 Marcia Mulloy
Thumbnail photo on back cover by Leah LaBar

The information, ideas, and suggestions in this book are not intended as a substitute
for professional medical advice. Neither the author nor the publisher shall be
liable or responsible for any loss or damage allegedly arising as a consequence of
your use or application of any information or suggestions in this book.
While many of the concepts and techniques are simple, human experiences
can be complex. Study with an experienced practitioner is advised.

iUniverse books may be ordered through booksellers or by contacting:

iUniverse
1663 Liberty Drive
Bloomington, IN 47403
www.iuniverse.com
1-800-Authors (1-800-288-4677)

Because of the dynamic nature of the Internet, any web addresses or links contained in
this book may have changed since publication and may no longer be valid. The views
expressed in this work are solely those of the author and do not necessarily reflect the
views of the publisher, and the publisher hereby disclaims any responsibility for them.

Any people depicted in stock imagery provided by Thinkstock are models,
and such images are being used for illustrative purposes only.
Certain stock imagery © Thinkstock.

ISBN: 978-1-4917-9922-2 (sc)
ISBN: 978-1-4917-9923-9 (hc)
ISBN: 978-1-4917-9924-6 (e)

Library of Congress Control Number: 2016909572

Print information available on the last page.

iUniverse rev. date: 07/12/2016

Fiction books by Mary Szczepanski

A Path of Healing by Mary Z

Megan is a troubled thirteen-year-old when she is sent from her family in New York City to stay with her eccentric aunt in southeast Alaska. On a challenging wilderness adventure she unexpectedly discovers her healing abilities. (2013)

Strands

This fiction book tells the story of Maya, and her life as a reluctant healer in a future where humans are evolving more DNA and more physical and mental abilities. As Maya and her closest friends in Albuquerque, New Mexico, work to make the world a better place, she finds that her own fate is tied to the evolution of everyone on earth. (2014)

CONTENTS

Illustrations and credits

Figure 1 Marcia Mulloy
Figure 2 Layout Patti Restaino, figure Marcia Mulloy
Figure 3 Zara Sykes and Marcia Mulloy
Figure 4 Zara Sykes and Marcia Mulloy
Figure 5 Marcia Mulloy
Thumbnail photo on back cover by Leah LaBar

While many of the concepts and techniques are simple, human experiences can be complex. Study with an experienced practitioner is advised.

PREFACE

I have always believed in miracles. Though most experiences of being raised in an organized religion are distant memories, the realm of the wondrous and supernatural continues to resonate deeply in my soul. From a young age I knew there was more than the material world, more to people than flesh and bones, and I never needed proof of the invisible pathways by which things happened. I didn't know *how* miracles were possible, but from the first moment of learning about these unseen forces, I knew that they were as true as anything that could be seen or touched. Decades later, I still wonder why people aren't more excited about them.

In the early years my only access to miracles was to wish for certain things to happen … getting a certain grade, going on important outings of youth, wanting my father to quit drinking. Even praying hard was like a form of spiritual roulette. Maybe something happened, maybe it didn't.

Meandering along life's pathway I caught glimpses of a reality beyond the obvious. It was like seeing light through the opening of a mysterious door, just barely ajar. Over a lifetime there have been many *peak experiences*: exhilarating moments or flashes of a connection to a life beyond this life, though nearly all were disappointingly fleeting.

As an undergraduate in nursing school in New York City in the early 70's, I went to a yoga class taught by two men from India in turbans and robes. The class took place in a hotel room with the beds removed. There were only a handful of students. We practiced just three to five postures in an hour, holding them for several minutes with great focus, then resting in between, and then repeating the sequence. I could feel the movement of energy and healing through my muscles; peacefulness permeated my consciousness.

Yoga was relatively new to the West. On one visit to my family in Buffalo, New York, I showed them some simple postures I had learned. They thought it was hilarious: some "far out" practice just too bizarre for the average person. Yet ironically, one of my sisters later started a yoga practice and the other began studies and practice in Qi Gong, another type of energy work.

While still in nursing school at Cornell Medical Center, I participated in a small meditation group. We were seated on the floor cross-legged in silence. Within minutes of a gentle breathing exercise, I experienced a bright white light that seemed to be coming from within me. Though brief it was quite profound — one of those peak experiences that stayed in my awareness and surfaced at intervals throughout my life. I later learned that this was very likely a *Kundalini* experience in which energy travels up the spine to awaken consciousness, resulting in a blissful state.

In the mid 1970's I moved to Durango, Colorado, a beautiful town nestled next to the La Plata Mountains and Animas River. It was a paradise of sunshine, hiking, skiing in winter, and more opening to spirit. The day I arrived in Durango I drove past a fast food restaurant on the main street. The sign in front read "Howdy, Mary!" Whether a coincidence or a miracle I took it as a *sign* that moving there was the right choice.

In addition to the outdoor activities and the environment of Durango, there were healers, teachers and friends who helped me travel further into the realm of the sacred. One friend, Judy, shared books by Godfré Ray King. The books described the *I Am* teachings channeled from Count Saint Germain, an alchemist, who allegedly lived for hundreds of years. There were stories of beings so well aligned with Source energy that they could precipitate food and other objects directly from the atmosphere. Judy and I also went to a gifted psychotherapist, Therese, for a few dream interpretation sessions. We would each take some guesses at the meaning of our own and each other's dream, and then Therese would tap into her vast store of Jungian symbolism and share more possibilities. It was always enlightening. I was most relieved to learn that my dream about putting my own dead body into a drawer was likely a metaphor for changes in my life at the time and not my impending death.

Before moving to Durango, I was getting a lift from some friendly people in Buffalo. A young man showed me a book he was reading called *Seth Speaks*. Although the book contained topics that interested me and the individual was wildly enthusiastic about the book, the title put me off and I did not pursue it any further. After moving to Durango some time later, I was visiting new friends. As I walked through their front door, I was stopped in front of the bookshelf right near the entrance as if by an invisible force. Just at eye level, *Seth Speaks* was sticking out of the row of books. I could not walk past the bookcase without asking to borrow it. I felt a warm, comforting intuitive sense that it was the right time to read the book. And so it was!

Seth Speaks records the channeled words of the being, Seth, spoken through Jane Roberts and recorded by her husband. The book reports dramatic scenes of groups of people getting psychic information, ideas about consciousness, and the possibilities of other realities. While reading the book, I had a dream during which I was able to see the electromagnetic energy in my hand and forearm. I was awed by the movement of colors and the harmonious musical vibrations emanating from within my arm in a dynamic and mystical choreography.

This book left me wanting more. I readily studied whatever was available: *Touch for Health* (meridian work), Tai Chi with Dolores La Chapelle, and *A Course in Miracles* (a spiritual teaching of universal love and peace). I went to a one week seminar on Imagery, which focused on using the power of the imagination for healing. At the annual Science of Mind conference, I heard Marilyn Ferguson speak about *The Aquarian Conspiracy*; Buckminster Fuller shared a vision for accessing unlimited potential of the mind; and Jean Houston talked about the *Possible Human*. Dorothy Maclean, a founder of the Findhorn community in Scotland, described the community's spiritual and ecological endeavors in northern Scotland. With the help of nature spirits, and against the odds — poor soil, harsh climate — they built a successful and sustainable agriculture project that is now a U.N. education center and continues to be mostly self-supporting. Thirty years later, I visited Findhorn which is now home to hundreds of people, much larger than Dorothy described in the early 1980's. All these ideas were exhilarating for me and motivated me to keep learning more.

In 1985 I moved from Durango to Denver for graduate school at the University of Colorado to study Community Health Nursing. In Denver I met the late Janet Mentgen, founder of Healing Touch, which is now an international course of study. I was fortunate to have Janet as a nurse entrepreneur preceptor for a graduate school requirement. In the 1980's her classes were just beginning. Janet taught Yoga Nidra (psychic sleep) meditation, biofeedback, and courses that eventually evolved into Healing Touch. Janet supported students with her leadership and encouraged us to teach Healing Touch when we were ready, as well as other classes reflecting many of our interests and skills. As a result the growing support community was exposed to numerous vibrational healing methods. For example, one nurse, Dona L., was a tremendous resource for body-mind healing. She once brought in a man who used copper tubing to form the outlines of three-dimensional platonic solids. Each copper structure was large enough to sit in and each gave off specific vibrations. The pyramid was popular for meditation, but my lasting memory was sitting in the dodecahedron, a twelve-sided figure. It made my heart race until I felt forced to get out of it, which convinced me that shapes do hold frequencies and that frequencies have an effect on a person. I was introduced to Axiatonal Grid Work and the Mari-El vibration which further expanded my awareness of energy healing. More recently I learned a bioscalar technique and a bit of polarity.

At one energy healing class, we used finger sticks to take blood samples from each other. We examined red blood cells under a microscope before and after energy work. Before the treatments, some of the cells would stick together in a "stacked" formation. After treatments, the cells were nearly all separate and moving freely – an improved state for oxygen and carbon dioxide exchange.

It was wonderful to share space with Janet in the office suite. I gave treatments and helped several instructors write objectives for nurses' continuing education, which involved translating esoteric concepts into clear learning objectives.

Healing Touch has been the central modality in my private practice. I have taught Healing Touch and holistic classes in twelve locations in Alaska where I currently live, over a dozen states in the U.S, as well as Canada, Romania, Ireland, U.K., and introductions in Poland.

I often use the Emotional Freedom Technique or EFT, which involves tapping acupressure meridians to re-balance the energy field, for myself and my clients. I teach Healing Touch Levels 1-5, and other energy related classes, including Healing Trauma and Pain Management with Holistic Approaches. I am now a Reiki master. I continue to do some nursing on a psychiatric unit as well as coordinate Healing Touch for patients and staff at the local hospital. I enjoy teaching holistic health skills to patients there, especially on the addictions recovery unit, as well as in the community.

My experiences with various spiritual communities and with energy work have helped me to keep moving closer to my true self. It seems there is a place within each of us that allows us to know what is true. If undamaged, that part of us acts as the compass that guides us through stormy waters or keeps us in tune with the rhythms of life. I believe it is that inner guidance that has brought me to the awareness of miracles and energy healing and continues to inspire me on the quest toward higher consciousness.

ACKNOWLEDGEMENTS

I would like to thank all my teachers, especially the late Janet Mentgen, as well as my clients, students, friends, and family who have inspired me, contributed their stories, and supported me in writing this book. Thanks to my sister, Margie Szczepanski for the gift which made possible the professional editing. Special thanks to Marcia Mulloy for much feedback and helping with numerous artistic and technical tasks; and to Marsha Buck, Linni Esther, Kay Havely, Lisa Bell, Marcia Mulloy, and others for proofreading. I would like to extend my deepest thanks to all of you and to Sue Behnert, Darcy Lockhart, Judy Macnack, Leah LaBar, Julie DeLong, Nanci Moore, and the many others who offered encouragement all along the way.

INTRODUCTION

This book is not a scientific document or research report. My purpose in writing it is to share my experiences, and a few simple techniques in hopes that they will open a door for others to explore energy healing and its applications, and give readers an opportunity to move more deeply into their own wholeness and discover their own miracles.

The book begins by providing some working definitions of holistic approaches and energy healing with various examples of different types of energy work, followed by a comparison of Western and Holistic approaches. There is a description of the energy field and basic techniques, preparation suggestions for doing energy work, examples of client responses, and some principles of ethical behavior when working with clients. Then the all-important self care and meditation for energy workers is addressed. Special situations such as life transitions, trauma, and distance healing are each given a separate chapter, followed by types of personal transformation that can occur as a result of giving or receiving energy healing. The final chapter pulls together historical background information, science and examples of related research in order to show how energy healing came to be relevant in current times and to help anchor the material presented in daily life.

CHAPTER 1

OPENING THE DOOR
TO HEALING

Energy Healing

Healing can be defined as restoring health, or the act of making whole. Energy healing is a simple, non-invasive way to restore balance to the human energy field to enhance the functioning of the body and increase a sense of well-being. When balance is achieved, a person may feel more whole and more connected with themselves and others. Energy healing generally results in relaxation and often brings clarity of thought and relief of symptoms.

Energy healing is done by medical professionals as well as lay people from all walks of life. There are many types of energy healing techniques available. Some approaches involve working with acupuncture meridians and points, or reflexology areas of the hands and feet that balance the energy of the body. For example, the Brazilian Toe technique involves holding the toes in a specific sequence to achieve a healing effect. Energy healing sessions such as Healing Touch use specific techniques with light touch or no touch to clear and balance the energy field and energy centers, while holding a positive intention for healing. An interesting aspect of Healing Touch and some other energy healing techniques is that the practitioner and client needn't be in the same physical location to work together. Sessions can be done remotely, where the giver and receiver are in two completely different locations.

Energy healing can be done on oneself or on another person (the client). It can also be done by two or more people working on a client. Energy healing is convenient and generally requires no special equipment. It can be done in professional or casual settings. It may be used to prevent illness or when someone is injured, or becomes ill suddenly, after he or she is physically stabilized.

Healing Touch can be used in combination with other medicinal approaches, such as medication, or before and after medical procedures, and often boosts the effectiveness of these methods. Some massage therapists use energy work before and after the massage, so that the effects of the massage will last longer. Healing Touch helps to reduce side effects of medical treatment and can greatly reduce complications from an illness or injury. Here are a few examples of how I've used Healing Touch.

A woman requested Healing Touch for sciatica, a painful nerve inflammation condition. Chiropractic treatments had relieved the pain, but the result did not last long. In the Healing Touch treatment, she received a specific sequence of techniques for treating back pain. Following the treatment she was free of pain for three months.

A nurse friend had gall bladder surgery. Following the surgery she was experiencing a high level of nausea, which the anesthesiologist predicted. With her permission I cleared her energy field with a non-contact Healing Touch technique until she reported that she was no longer nauseated.

Another friend, Sara, was having her wisdom teeth removed. I suggested she try Healing Touch before and after the surgery to help reduce swelling. The first treatment was the day prior to surgery, the second was within an hour after the teeth were pulled. As Sara described it, "It was so soothing. I remember kind of just drifting off. And you know — I didn't have any swelling. It was so great!"

Once while traveling on a plane, the flight attendants called for medical help. A woman was travelling home after having had a hip replacement and thought she dislocated the hip as she settled into her seat shortly after take-off.

As a psychiatric nurse I hesitated to respond, but knew I could at least offer comfort with energy healing techniques. The woman was very anxious and extremely uncomfortable. I asked if she wanted to try Healing Touch for pain relief and relaxation. She had taken some ibuprofen, but was still tense and frightened. She agreed to let me do some Healing Touch. She was in the aisle seat; her husband gave me the middle seat and he moved to the window. I spent the next hour clearing the energy at her hip. She was able to relax and was less frightened. Healing Touch may have also helped the ibuprofen to be more effective for pain relief.

A healer named Richard Gordon videotaped energy healing classes he taught called *Quantum Touch*:

He showed that even beginning students using Quantum Touch could have an effect. In one class students assessed each other's spinal alignment by comparing the level of the hips while standing. Even after a brief session, students could see the alignment of the spine improved as evidenced by the hips becoming more level.

As with many other experiences in life, the effects of energy healing are influenced by relationship, specifically the quality of the relationship between the giver and the receiver. A trusting relationship will help both parties to feel safe and allow the energy to move more easily.

Energy healing requires no particular belief and is not affiliated with any religion, although many religions have had healing as a part of their framework. When healing is part of a religious practice it is often a type of healing called *faith healing*, where a belief in the religion is important in order for the healing to work. In energy healing it is not necessary for an individual to believe that energy healing will work, but negative attitudes about the healing can block the effects of it. Healthy skepticism does not create resistance as long as one is open to the possibility that energy healing can have a desirable effect.

While some individuals have a natural "gift" for doing healing work, it is a skill that can be learned. Practitioners and recipients alike find that energy healing can help them "tune in" to the subtle forces in and around them. The more we practice skills, the more sensitive we also become to our intuitive abilities.

Energy healing is evolving as underlying principles and our understanding of those principles changes over time. In many schools of healing, only the mind is needed to influence the changes needed to affect healing. Perhaps the energy healing of the future will be done only with the mind.

Effects of Energy Healing

The effects of energy healing can occur on the physical, emotional, mental, and/or spiritual (PEMS) levels:

- **Physical**: Relaxation is the most common experience during or after Healing Touch. Often there is at least some relief of pain or other physical symptoms.

    There was a male patient in the hospital after a stroke. He was unable to progress to rehabilitation services until he could swallow. I had given him two Healing Touch treatments, which helped him relax and feel better, but he still could not swallow. He and his wife had an interest in alternative healing and he responded well to the first treatments. For the third treatment, I decided to use a more potent technique based on the work of Barbara Brennan. That night not only was he was able to swallow, but he was moved to rehab services the next day to continue his healing process. It was not possible to determine whether the change was due to the cumulative effect of three sessions or his own resilience, but I was glad to have contributed my skills for whatever benefit they may have provided.

- **Emotional**: Emotional responses to energy healing can be quite profound. Common emotional experiences include feelings such as love, peace, joy, or releasing feelings such as grief, sadness, or anger.

    A nurse called me to the hospital to offer Healing Touch to a patient who was upset and angry after talking to her doctor. The patient had had bariatric (stomach reduction) surgery for extreme obesity. During the Healing Touch treatment she relaxed deeply and dozed off. When I finished she was cheerful and grateful for the treatment.

- **Mental**: Increased mental clarity is a common result of energy healing. Clarity might include gaining a new understanding of an issue, resolving a conflict, or changing an attitude or behavior. O. Carl Simonton said in his book *Getting Well Again,* "In order to get well, you have to learn to think in a new way. "

At a health fair, one of the individuals who signed up for a brief treatment was a high school female who was going to play basketball that afternoon. I hesitated to give her a treatment at first, thinking it might make her too relaxed to play well. I saw her on the street a few weeks later. She reported that after Healing Touch she was able to score some points in the game, which she had never done before. Perhaps the energy work cleared self doubt that was in the way of performing with confidence.

A male WWII veteran sustained many injuries from the war, including shrapnel, loss of one eye, and chronic pain. He regularly saw a doctor at a clinic. The nurses there reported that he was consistently in pain and hostile toward them whenever he came in for an appointment. However, he agreed to receive Healing Touch when it was offered by the nurses as something that might help him. After a number of treatments the nurses reported that although he continued to have pain and numerous medical problems, he was no longer aggressive toward the staff.

- **Spiritual:** There is an energy field that spans the universe and permeates all things, connecting us to all of existence. Spirituality may be found in feeling a connection to the energy of a Higher Power or in finding a sense of meaning and purpose in life. These feelings may emerge after an energy healing session. Occasionally, some have experienced a meeting with a Higher Power or divine beings or spiritual guidance.

One female patient, in the hospital for respiratory problems, reported seeing angels during the Healing Touch treatment.

Once at a Healing Touch conference participants were sharing some of their experiences. A Jewish man described how all his life he felt he was carrying the tremendous weight of the historical oppression experienced by Jewish people. After one treatment, even though he knew that anti-Semitism had not ended, he felt the heavy weight of it lifted from his own energy field.

Some General Applications for Energy Healing

Increased vitality	When congested energy is released and the energy field is balanced, a person is likely to feel more alive and energized.
Stress management	Having a balanced energy field helps an individual to feel more mentally and emotionally resilient and able to cope with life's stresses. With practice, relaxation can be maintained even during stress.
Mental clarity	Disorganized, scattered, or unfocused thinking can improve when the energy field is balanced and grounded.
Restful sleep	The deep relaxation of energy healing can promote healthy, restorative sleep.
Prevention of illness	A balanced energy field promotes the body's natural healing ability, including boosting the immune system.
Pain relief	Energy healing can be used for acute or chronic pain, including headache, back, joint, muscle, or organ pain. It can increase the effectiveness of pain medications and other treatments.

Healing of illness, injuries, or symptoms	Since energy healing promotes the body's natural ability to heal, it may speed healing from various ailments as well as minimize complications.
Emotional healing	Healing Touch helps release anger, resentments, grief, and the effects of trauma.
Care of the sick	Energy healing provides comfort when pain relief is not possible, and may help a person feel whole when recovery is not likely. One can create a healing environment by clearing the energy in the room, and energizing medications, linens, bandages, or food.
Comfort for the dying	A healing presence provides comfort for dying individuals or their family members, assisting them to a peaceful transition.
Release of toxins	Healing Touch can provide an energetic detox from ingested substances, pollution, environmental toxins, or even emotional toxins.
Addictions recovery	Besides helping in an energetic detox, energy healing can help release emotional baggage, clarify thinking, and increase spiritual awareness. Rebalancing the energy centers, especially the connection between heart and mind is often critical for addictions recovery. EFT can release cravings and many symptoms and underlying causes of addiction.
Dealing with the unknown	Energy healing helps one to connect with internal resources and stay balanced during trying times.
Challenging or chaotic social situations	Holding a high vibration during challenging social events may bring harmony and possibly contribute to a more positive outcome, whether at a party, a political event, an environmental crisis, or during international unrest.

| Spiritual connection and intuitive abilities. | Staying energetically balanced brings peace of mind, opens awareness to deeper intuition, and maintains alignment with Source energy. |

CHAPTER 2

WESTERN MEDICINE AND HOLISTIC PRACTICE

Western Medicine v. Holistic Healing

Western or allopathic medicine is different from Holistic Healing in several ways. Western medicine uses medication and surgery to relieve specific symptoms or cure conditions. These treatments can often be completed quickly and produce immediate results. As such, allopathic medicine may be the best choice for life-threatening conditions or situations in which an organ or limb is in serious danger.

The cost of Western medicine is usually reimbursed by a third party insurer who may monetarily exert an influence on the treatment provided. For example, a cardiologist might receive little or no insurance reimbursement for teaching a patient about making lifestyle choices that will improve his or her condition. However, the same cardiologist might receive a moderate reimbursement for performing an angioplasty, and a huge payment for more complicated heart surgery. The patient agrees to the treatment, takes medication or submits to the procedure, and may need to do some follow-up (e.g. physical therapy exercises) that is also reimbursed. The focus in this scenario is on physical recovery. Spiritual insights, emotional healing, and personal transformation are typically not addressed in Western medical practice.

Holistic health refers to the care of the whole person: body, mind, and spirit. Holistic practice promotes and values the active participation of the patient in his or her treatment. Thus the patient is more active in their care. The patient or client is often encouraged to take responsibility for changing one or more behaviors in order to be healthier. Holistic healing is often an effective approach to chronic illnesses which tend to require lifestyle changes in order for symptoms to improve or be prevented. Over time and with proper treatment and attention, clients can achieve positive results physically, mentally, emotionally, or spiritually.

Interestingly, some well-known healers have reported that the main cause of their own illness was that they were *not being true to their soul.* Hildegarde of Bingen, an 11th century mystic, was ill and fatigued until she accepted her calling to teach and help others. Brugh Joy, MD described stomach problems which affected him until he surrendered to his inner guidance to do holistic work. This concept of living a life true to one's self is rarely if ever addressed in Western medicine, yet it seems to be one of the central concepts tying together many holistic traditions. In holistic theory and practice, the components of one's life and work are integrated and have an effect on one's health.

Here is a summary of some of the differences between the two approaches to medicine and health:

<u>Western/ Allopathic Medicine</u>	<u>Holistic Healing/ Integrative medicine</u>
Goal is the cure or relief symptoms.	Focus is on wholeness and balance, and integration of body, mind, and spirit. Goal may also be personal transformation.
Works best on acute, life threatening conditions.	Addresses lifestyle changes needed to prevent illness or manage chronic conditions. Treats stress.

Medication, surgery and radiation are the main approaches.	Uses a wide range of body/mind approaches: diet/nutrition, supplements, breathing and relaxation exercises, meditation, energy work, imagery/self hypnosis, movement (e.g. yoga, tai chi), bodywork, journaling, homeopathic remedies.
Death is often considered a failure and huge amounts of money are spent to prevent it. Death is often accepted only when "nothing more can be done".	Death is part of the life cycle. Approaches may focus on comfort, acceptance, and a peaceful transition.
Practitioner owns knowledge and performs most of the actions needed to "fix" the problem.	Client is more often a partner and often commits to making changes in behavior to improve health. Client is encouraged to have knowledge for self care.
Costs are often reimbursed and can be influenced by third party payers (insurance companies).	As of this writing, holistic modalities are usually self-pay, although corporations often see the value of health promotion for employees and may offer free programs. Public health projects promote self care, including healthy eating, exercising 60 minutes/day, stress management, etc. Supported programs may be free or have reduced rates.
Quantitative research methods are used to show efficacy of many techniques.	Qualitative research addresses quality of life issues. More quantitative research is also being done.

Describes cause and effect in linear time. Time for resolution of symptoms from known illnesses is often predicted.	May see time as simultaneous. Healing can happen instantly and is not dependent on linear time. Personal transformation may be the work of a lifetime.
Seeks physical causes for physical problems.	Causes can be physical, emotional, mental, spiritual, social, environmental, or combinations of these.

CHAPTER 3

THE HUMAN ENERGY FIELD: LEVELS AND ENERGY CENTERS

Levels of the Field

The energy field has been called the *aura,* though scientists more commonly refer to it as the *biofield* or bio-electro-magnetic field. This energy field exists in and around the body and functions to hold and exchange information. Energy itself is a neutral force, though energy fields can influence each other. Janet Mentgen, in years of teaching Healing Touch, would say: "Energy has no opinion, no belief, and no attitude."

The energy field is an open system in which energy can flow in and out. Ideally healthy, life-affirming energy is absorbed, and disruptive influences flow out. Energy healing positively influences the energy field to become more clear and balanced.

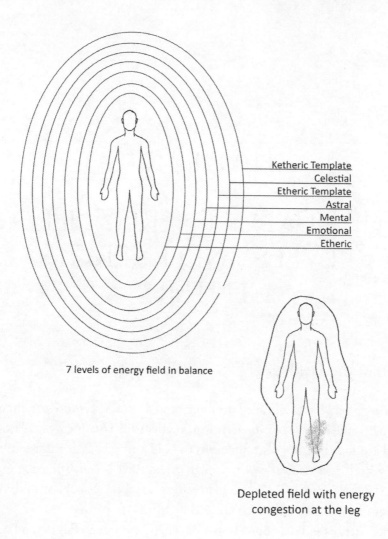

Ketheric Template
Celestial
Etheric Template
Astral
Mental
Emotional
Etheric

7 levels of energy field in balance

Depleted field with energy
congestion at the leg

Figure 1

When balanced, energy within and around the body is a dynamic field in which the energy flows freely and purposefully to maintain health for the body, mind, and spirit. Its radius extends to an arm's distance around the body and might be seen or felt as an egg shape. Many models and theories about the energy field exist. Keep in mind that the field is more dynamic than a drawing or even a three dimensional model can portray.

In her book *Hands of Light* (1988), Barbara Brennan gives names to the levels of the field: *etheric* (related to the physical body), *emotional* (emotions), *mental* (thoughts and attitudes), *astral* (compassion and forgiveness), *etheric template* (energetic blueprint), *celestial* (intuitive), and *ketheric template* (spiritual). Each level permeates the body and the other levels, and extends further from the body than the previous one. Each level has a higher frequency than the one preceding it. Because the energy is a subtle force, the different levels are also referred to as *subtle bodies*.

Disturbances and Rebalancing

A balanced field supports life processes (See Figure 1). Illness results when the flow of energy is short-circuited. Areas affected by the disruption hold a low vibration which can cause illness, immune problems, or other symptoms (Figure 1). These disrupted areas might be detected visually by some healers, or more commonly felt as "congestion" in the field. An unbalanced energy field can make someone feel emotionally unstable, take on a negative or angry attitude, or feel spiritually disconnected. Energy balancing techniques can help people feel better about themselves and promote peacefulness and positive action toward others in the world.

The process of energy healing raises the vibration of disrupted or congested areas so that they are in balance with the rest of the field. In cases where the entire field is depleted, energy healing can increase the vibration of the whole field. When the vibration of the entire field is raised, balanced, and energized with or without the help of a healer a person's natural healing abilities function better. Energy healing is self-healing.

Since energy follows thought, the mind can be used to re-balance the field. However, this also works in the opposite sense, as negative thoughts, worry, fear, and anxiety have low vibrations and can create imbalances that leave the field vulnerable. Energy workers attempt to re-balance the energy field by using their hands near the body or lightly touching the body, while holding a healing intention.

Energy fields can influence each other. For example, a person with an upbeat attitude can emit positive energy and help others to feel more positive. Some popular celebrities and gurus have large energy fields that attract fans or followers. The process of one field influencing another is called *induction*. When one field is influenced by another, the affected field is said to become entrained with the vibration of the other.

Energy Centers

There are seven major energy centers called *chakras* in the human body. Chakra is a Sanskrit word meaning "wheel of light." Each major chakra is a funnel-shaped spinning vortex and each vortex has a different frequency and therefore a different color. Each major chakra energizes an area of the body, usually the area in the immediate vicinity of its location. It also energizes a major nerve plexus and an endocrine gland. There are minor chakras (minor energy centers) throughout the joints and organs. Note: Knowledge about energy fields and chakras comes from many traditions and through the perceptions of many individuals. Perhaps this accounts for variations in the descriptions in different resources.

Major Chakras

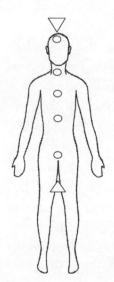

	Name	Area	Gland	Issue
7 Violet	Crown	Upper Brain	Pineal	Spiritual
6 Indigo	Brow	Lower Brain	Pituitary	Intuition
5 Azure	Throat	Lungs, Throat	Thyroid, Para Thyroid	Creativity, Expression
4 Green	Heart	Heart, Blood, Circulation, Chest	Thymus	Compassion
3 Yellow	Solar Plexus	Digestive system	Pancreas	Mental
2 Orange	Sacral	Reproduction	Gonads	Emotional
1 Red	Root	Kidneys, Feet, Legs Spinal column	Adrenals	Survival, Will to live

Figure 2

Each chakra corresponds with a different level of the energy field. The first chakra corresponds with the etheric level, the second with the mental, and so on.

Carolyn Myss teaches that chakras maintain the energy field and can change energy from one frequency to another, like a metaphoric transformer. She described this flow of energy when one receives an inspiration: The energy begins at the crown chakra (7th chakra) and progresses through the chakras as the idea takes shape and the individual begins planning (6th), expresses creativity (5th), becomes more passionate about it (4th), puts willpower behind it and makes a commitment to it (3rd), feels emotionally connected to it (2nd), and manifests the idea on the material plane (1st). In this way the chakras are transformers of the energy, changing spiritual energy to intuitive energy, to passion and commitment, and continuing until the inspiration becomes reality. Withdrawing interest from a project or pulling back out of fear takes energy away from successful completion.

Chakras that are depleted or out of balance have a low vibration. They do not provide energy needed by the field and instead will hold the energy disturbances or low frequencies of injury or illness. Energy healing can release these disturbances, rebalance the field, raise the frequencies, and promote healing.

A friend came to my home requesting a Healing Touch treatment. As part of the treatment I was balancing her chakras. Each time I changed hand positions on the major chakras, she began sobbing. She explained that at each chakra she had a different memory of being abused. I asked if she wanted me to stop. She told me to continue, and that she could feel the emotional releases needed for healing as the chakras re-balanced. After releasing these traumatic emotions she felt more peaceful.

Much more information is available from other sources about the energy field and chakras. The basic description in this book is intended as a usable framework to help the reader apply the simple techniques described in chapters 5 and 6.

CHAPTER 4

PREPARATION: ENVIRONMENT, ENERGY WORKER, AND CLIENTS

In doing energy healing, certain preparations enhance the quality of the treatment and maintain safety in the environment. A relaxed energy worker in a pleasant environment will help the client relax. If the client knows what to expect it will be easier for them to be receptive.

Preparing the Environment

Creating a Peaceful Setting. Ideally it is comforting for a client to receive energy healing in a setting that is nurturing, quiet, free of clutter, and free of disturbances from phones or other noise. Some energy healers have a space particularly designed with soothing colors and décor that promotes restfulness and peace.

At times it may be desirable to clear the energy of the space being used. Although some might burn sage or light a candle, one can use intention to clear a room of any energy that was previously there, particularly if the room was used for a different purpose. State out loud or in one's mind, "This space is clear of previous energy and is now a *healing space*." Allow the healing energy of the universe or Source energy to flow through you and expand into all parts of the room where you are giving a treatment, teaching, or even having meetings.

When planning space for energy healing work, be aware that each person has specific needs. While aromas and music work well for some, others have allergies to *any* fragrances (even high quality products used for aromatherapy) and many people prefer quiet instead of music so that they can listen within.

Opportunities to provide energy healing may also occur in busy places, or when fear, anxiety, an injury, or sudden illness has occurred. In these situations, creating a healing space could be done by establishing rapport with the person in need of treatment, introducing oneself, asking permission to do energy work, and using intention. The energy fields of the client and energy worker can form a container or "bubble" for the healing work, even when the location is public or chaotic or filled with medical equipment. Small or symbolic adjustments can be made to help set the intention, such as rearranging furniture or other objects to identify and delineate the sacred space.

I've noticed at health fairs how volunteers invite a recipient to sit down, often after subtly moving the chair a hardly perceptible distance. It is as if the first position of the chair was quite ordinary, but after being moved, it becomes a healing space.

Safety. In any situation where energy work is performed, safety is a most important element, and this includes both physical and emotional safety. If the client is initially in an unsafe situation, remove the danger or remove the client from the situation if possible. Administer necessary first aid, get help if needed, and manage the emergency. Once all has been done in that regard, the energy work can begin, and may help reduce bleeding and swelling and help stabilize and comfort the client while awaiting further assistance.

In non-emergency situations, physical safety includes keeping furniture, such as a chair or massage table, in good working condition and arranging it for access and comfort e.g. a small step stool can help clients get on and off a massage table. Clear away shoes or other objects from around the table to avoid tripping. If the client will be offered water after a treatment, have it available before you begin treatment. See Addendum A for additional suggestions.

Energy healing is performed with giver and receiver fully clothed, with shoes being optional. Massage therapists using energy work will have the client properly draped.

Emotional safety is provided by developing rapport through listening — without giving advice or being judgmental. Every person wants to be seen, heard, appreciated, and understood for who they are. The focus of the interaction should be on the client's needs, carefully observing agreements about time and about remuneration if there is any. Ethical practice also dictates that the energy worker refers clients for treatment to other licensed professionals if the client has a condition or request beyond the energy worker's skills or scope of practice.

Preparation for the Energy Worker

Self-awareness. Those who are giving energy treatments need to be mentally and emotionally stable enough so as not to have a distracting or disturbing impact on the client, or be triggered by the client's issues or emotions. The energy worker should be sufficiently aware of his or her own issues to avoid projecting them onto the client.

I received two effective back treatments from the same energy practitioner. In the first session, she perceived that I had some problems with my mother, though receiving this type of "reading" was not a part of the work described. I wasn't aware of problems with my mother. In the next session, I was given the same unsolicited information, and suspected that the practitioner had problems with her own mother.

In energy healing, the worker often taps into a meditation state or an expanded state of consciousness that is useful in tuning in to subtle energy. The discipline needed for energy assessments and allowing energy to move through one's energy field often shifts the brain to use its alpha, theta, delta, or possibly more recently discovered gamma states. Although referred to as altered states, these are natural states that occur spontaneously with day dreaming, using the imagination, sleep cycles, meditation, or other focused activities. However, the energy worker needs to be aware of these states and maintain a focus on the client.

Mentorship. Some people may be born with special abilities, but many approaches to healing can be learned. Although numerous energy techniques are simple and easily applied, there is a great benefit in studying with experienced practitioners. These masters can help guide us through clinically and ethically challenging situations and encourage a novice through his or her spiritual development.

Intention. In energy healing it is best to maintain an intention for the *highest good,* beyond the condition for which a treatment is requested. The clients might have unknown needs or needs they do not feel comfortable sharing. A client may request work for a physical complaint when the real need is psychological or spiritual. For example, it may be easier for a client to say he has back pain than to share that he lost his job, that his partner is leaving, or that he feels his life is in shambles. A broad intention that focuses on the client's highest good will encompass whatever is needed, including unspoken hopes and issues beyond awareness. Setting an intention for the highest good also reminds us that we are not in control, but that as healers we are surrendering to the Source of the energy. (Note: Occasionally questions arise about whether energy healing could be used for a negative purpose. However, intentions to cause harm are not energy healing.)

Healing Presence. Whether or not we are able to provide hands-on energy treatments, we can have a positive effect on various situations by being aware in the moment and holding an intention. Some refer to this as *holding the light.* Others around us may respond to this healing presence as their energy fields begin to resonate at a higher vibration. Holding a vibration of peace and caring can improve many situations, and is especially helpful when the client is fearful or when the environment is chaotic.

One can be a healing presence in all situations: a family meal, a meeting in the community or even during a phone conversation. Hearing a crash or an argument or an emergency siren can be used as an opportunity to expand our presence, and to hold a positive intention where needed. Even at the grocery store, a superficial transaction can be transformed into a meaningful interaction in a moment. A small amount of eye contact can create a notable feeling of "change" when monetary "change" is received from a clerk. Holding a positive, healing focus can help the healer develop and maintain a high vibration, as well as spread healing in the world.

Centering. Centering is aligning body, mind, and spirit, and is one of the most important aspects of preparation for healing work. Centering is the process of focusing one's attention in the present moment or going to an inner point of peace and maintaining it throughout the treatment. It is a process of releasing distractions and making oneself available for whatever needs to happen. Centering can improve decisions, interactions, and attitude. It enables healers to have the heightened awareness to be in touch with the flow of energy and use it as a guide for what needs to be balanced or released.

The quality of the healer's field will add to the effects of the healing technique and may provide greater impact than the techniques used. It is important for energy workers to develop the discipline to keep themselves balanced and at a high vibration. To be a clear channel for energy healing depends on releasing any possible obstructions, such as attitudes or symptoms within oneself. The ability to do energy healing is greatly improved with a regular meditation practice to clear the mind and maintain alignment with Source energy.

There are multiple opportunities for centering during a session: before the client arrives, before the assessment, before various techniques, or if attention drifts from the purpose of the session.

Centering can be done by using simple breathing exercises. For example, just focusing one's attention on the breath is a powerful tool to bring awareness to the moment. One can breathe in peacefulness and breathe out distractions. Usually several rounds are adequate to prepare oneself for giving an energy treatment. It is possible to shift one's awareness in just one breath. Think about how quickly a person can shift when answering the phone. Whether busy or upset, most people can answer with a congenial "hello" when prompted by the ring tone of the phone.

In a more advanced practice called *Tonglen* (from the Buddhist tradition), one can extend compassion for suffering and transform disharmony by breathing in the conflict and suffering of humanity and breathing out peacefulness — the opposite of the previously described breathing. In this practice, the heart is thought to transform the energy of suffering.

As I remember, Janet Mentgen, the founder of Healing Touch, suggested a brief centering, so as not to energetically distance oneself from the client's state. She thought that holding the client's hand, shoulders, or feet and setting the intention with them helps healer and client move forward together in the healing process.

Another common centering exercise is to visualize oneself as a tree. Feel the energy from the feet extending like roots going deep into the earth. Allow the healing energy from the earth to enter one's energy field from below. Then like the branches of a tree reaching upward bring in energy from the heavens above, allowing both forces to meet at the heart center.

Even without the tree image, the energy can be brought into one's field from the earth and the heavens and the four directions through intention. Allow the energy to meet at the heart center, move down the arms, and energize the hands for energy work.

Centering might involve connecting to the Source (the Source of All That Is, the Source of all healing, Higher Power, Divine Energy, Universal Healing Energy) and accessing this force to use in the healing process. Centering prevents taking on the client's issues. A healer does not give her or his own energy to the client — this would be exhausting. Instead, the healer connects with the unlimited universal healing energy, allowing that energy to clear and energize his or her own field, and then allows that energy flow to the client.

Allowing the healing energy to be channeled through one's energy field while giving a treatment creates a sense of wholeness and profound connection. This experience may feel more real than other life experiences because in accessing spiritual and intuitive abilities, we are detaching from ego-driven motives and being more authentic. It is generally a rewarding, fulfilling, and mutually transformative experience.

There is a book on my shelf called *Always Getting Ready*. It described the traditions of Yup'ik people of Alaska as they interact with the seasons and the cycles of nature. In healing work it is important to take care of one's own issues, to be open to the rhythm of life, and learn to release stuck patterns of energy while staying present for the challenges being experienced by clients. For energy workers, regular centering practices help maintain readiness for when healing skills are needed.

Grounding. The process of grounding is about connecting with the Earth energies through our feet to re-establish a sense of balance. For those raised in western religious beliefs, there is a tendency to think of the heavens above when accessing spirituality. However, if thoughts are focusing only upwards the rest of one's energy field can get out of balance. Rosalyn Bruyere, a contemporary healer and author, reminded students at a Healing Touch conference that the amount of energy that can be channeled through one's energy field is directly proportional to one's grounding. The term "grounding" is sometimes interchanged with the idea of centering, since both help bring one's awareness to the present moment.

Although it is rare, when things "go wrong" in a treatment, such as the healer becoming distracted, doubtful, confused, fearful, dizzy, forgetful about a technique, or experiencing the client's pain, these symptoms can generally be relieved by grounding to the Earth's energy field and remembering not to use one's personal energy for the treatment.

Grounding the client at the end of a session assures that they are alert and oriented to time and space. Here is an example of a failure to adequately ground a client:

I received a Gridwork treatment from an individual who was not grounded, as evidenced by the practitioner not being focused and chatting about different subjects during the treatment. Gridwork uses varying frequencies and dimensions to effect healing and transformation. There were a number of procedures at the end of the session requiring my attention and feedback, which were supposed to bring my awareness back. Yet when I got into my car after the session, I could not figure out how to turn on the ignition. Clearly, I was not sufficiently grounded to drive.

Grounding a client can be done by holding their feet or shoulders, offering them water to drink, or talking to them after the treatment. Asking about plans for the rest of the day brings a client out of the day dreaming state that might occur during or after the treatment and helps bring the client to an alert state. When the treatment is complete, grounding is a preparation for going back into the material world. If the client is a patient in the hospital, or will continue to sleep after the treatment, it is not necessary to bring them back to an alert state.

Attunement. Attuning is coming into relationship with the client's energy field and noting how the energy fields can meet for the best result. Attunement begins the flow of energy between the practitioner and client. It allows healers to tune into the deeper state of the person, not just the symptoms.

I recall and summarize the words of Janet Mentgen's suggestion for attuning:

Before you begin a treatment, take a moment to get a sense of the vibration of your energy field in relation to the client's energy field. Notice if your vibration is higher or lower than the client's. The healer will be most effective if his/her vibration is at a slightly higher frequency than the client's. If the healer's frequency is too low, he/she may not offer much to benefit the client. If his/her frequency is too high, the client may not be able to absorb the energy.

If one's vibration is lower than the client's, then one's energy can be increased in order to be effective. This can be done with intention, balancing one's chakras, or allowing more universal healing energy to move into one's field. If ones vibration is considerably higher than the client, intention can be used to create a vibration that is appropriately available to the client.

Let go of the outcome. Keep in mind that there are many unknowns about the effects of an energy session. The effects could occur physically, mentally, emotionally, or spiritually, regardless of the intention set. In general it is best to let go of expectations about outcomes and trust that there is some benefit, even though it may occur at a later time, or in a different way than expected, or not be observable.

Follow the Energy. Staying attuned during the session will make it possible to work with the client's energy as it shifts and changes. A client's need for pain relief may change to a need for emotional or mental clearing. A client's restlessness without other explanation can be a clue that something is making them uncomfortable. Sensing disruptions during an assessment may give additional information to where the energy field needs balancing. Janet Mentgen was known for saying, "Follow the energy", especially as it moves and changes.

Protection. Some energy workers have had concerns about "picking up symptoms" from a client. This is rarely an issue for experienced Healing Touch practitioners, when firmly grounded and connected with high vibration of Source energy. Keeping one's energy field clear and open allows for the release of anything taken in and not needed by one's own system. The release can be helped by intention, breathing, grounding, or self rebalancing of one's field. The energy field could be described as semi-permeable, rather than a barrier for protection which might prevent healing energy from flowing in or out.

Preparing the Client

First contact. An initial connection with the client may occur by phone or in person. How you ask questions and how you explain the work will demonstrate that you are safe and trustworthy. Each contact is an opportunity for a sacred exchange to take place. The first interaction is not just setting up an appointment, but might begin the process of a healing journey.

A Healing Relationship. Being gentle and kind will put most clients at ease and begin the process of relaxation. In a trusting relationship, clients will be more able to share their feelings, give feedback, and be partners in the healing work being done.

Eye contact when it is culturally and personally comfortable for clients can help clients feel they are receiving your attention. Find out what they know about energy healing and what goals they have for the treatment. Ask if they know what might be the cause of a problem, what remedies they have tried, or the meaning of a condition. They may already have accessed their inner wisdom.

Listening well is the best way to establish rapport. Being non-judgmental will help the client feel safe. Avoid giving advice or analyzing what the client shares. Being heard allows a person to process their experiences, think clearly, and make their own choices.

For a new client, be prepared to give a clear, simple definition of energy work in a few sentences. For those who have never experienced energy work, a short session or brief demonstration might help them understand what it is. Many people can only imagine this work as massage, so a demonstration may help clarify what will happen in a session.

Help the client to understand that the healer is a facilitator and as the energy field is balanced the client's body is doing the healing, noting that the process of healing might unfold in unexpected ways.

Explain how the treatment will be done, how long it will take, and what the client might expect, such as relaxation, peacefulness, or even occasionally increased pain before the pain is relieved. For example, *one nurse who received Healing Touch for cold symptoms stated that the symptoms became more intense but then cleared more quickly than she had anticipated, as if the process was speeded up.*

For some clients, the attention and caring given as the relationship is established can be healing in and of itself. It can open the process for trust, greater receptivity, and deeper healing.

Setting goals. Goals for a session should be clearly set before the treatment begins. Negotiating goals is another way to establish trust. The practitioner listens carefully to the client and helps them to set appropriate goals that are mutually agreeable. At times a desperate client may hope for a cure for a serious illness or immediate relief from a chronic debilitating condition. The terms *energy healing* and *Healing Touch* can misguide some to anticipate all-encompassing curative results, or care that is beyond the energy worker's skills. Being clear about what can be accomplished is important so that the client can have a choice about whether they want to consent to the treatment, or find other help. Cancer patients receiving chemotherapy might have less nausea and fatigue, as well as emotional and spiritual support, as a result of receiving Healing Touch. Pain may not be relieved, but the person might feel more whole and more accepting of his or her situation. A goal for relief of physical symptoms may not be met, but a client might get better sleep or experience a spiritual connection. Many are grateful for these results, even though a cure may not be available from energy healing. Energy workers can always help keep hope alive: hope to keep meaning and purpose in life, hope that symptoms will be manageable, and even hope that the client's own internal resources could help eliminate the illness.

Specific goals are easier to evaluate at the end of the treatment, e.g. headache relief, relaxation, feeling at peace. A very general goal such as "being a better person" might be too general to evaluate improvement after an hour session.

Intention. Give the client an opportunity, if he or she wishes, to verbalize an intention, or say it out loud for the client if it feels more comfortable. The intention (the agreed goal) may be to release pain, symptoms, emotional distress, or to gain mental clarity, a sense of peace and well-being, or any other intention the person might have in mind. Some feel that voicing the intention out loud helps creates a sound vibration to attract a healing resonance. Others might hold the intention silently.

Understanding Resistance. When doing any kind of personal work, the issue of psychological resistance sometimes arises. A client may initially deny any problems, even those which may be obvious to the observer, or may decline to begin or continue treatment. Although resistance is a protective mechanism to save a person from experiencing emotional pain, a client's denial, reluctance, fear, or belief can block the ability to get help or be receptive to energy healing. In energy work, allowing the resistance to surface without judgment can be the first step in energetically clearing it. For example, someone may want to quit smoking, but is afraid. Acknowledging the fear may help in clearing it energetically.

Sometimes a client will need to talk as part of their healing of grief or other deeply held emotions. At other times, constant talking may be part of a defense pattern that actually prevents the person from experiencing their feelings. This defense pattern is unconscious and openly discussing it might be outside the ability of the energy healer. Encouraging the client to relax quietly, but letting them know they can release any feelings that come up (crying, laughter, or expressing anger) during the treatment might assist them in healing emotions gently and safely.

Beliefs and opinions are forms of resistance that can block healing. If there is a large group belief creating an energy field that says the common cold will last seven to ten days, it could make it harder for people to heal more quickly. Carolyn Myss noted: "Healing can happen after years of therapy or after one good prayer." Acknowledging the possibilities of spontaneous remission, she remarked that healing can happen in the blink of an eye. When one's energy field is balanced and one's spirit is aligned with the Source, seemingly impossible things can happen. However, the recipient must be ready or at least open to receiving the healing. A dramatic change of this type sometimes requires a change in belief and lifestyle. Einstein is credited with saying "We can't solve problems by using the same kind of thinking we used when we created them."

Relaxation and Receptivity. Relaxation and a neutral or positive attitude about energy work can increase the receptivity of a client's energy field. Therefore, healing is more likely to occur when the client is relaxed. Taking the time to help the client get comfortable, whether sitting in a chair or lying on a massage table or other surface is worth the effort. Having someone get up after a session only to tell you they were uncomfortable the whole time is disappointing for both parties.

Some clients may need prompts or voice guiding for relaxation. Slowly talking them through relaxation from foot to head is simple and effective. You might use this sequence progressing slowly enough for one or more breaths for each body part to relax: "relax your feet…legs… pelvic area…now the abdomen… chest…spine…arms…now shoulders… neck…head…relax all the muscles in your face…." You can prompt the client to remember that with each breath the relaxation becomes deeper. Suggestions to feel the support of the table and release all tension, are useful. Let the client know they can move, change position, stretch, cough, or stop the treatment at any time for any reason, for example, if they are uncomfortable, or if the work is not what they expected.

I often encourage clients to let their mind take them to a vibration where all things are possible and all healing is available. In that vibration, they can set their intention for the session and absorb the healing energy of the universe for the highest good.

It might help to encourage the client to use the simple breathing exercise of paying attention to each breath. If they want to participate more, encourage them to put their awareness where your hands are, or to hold the intention of releasing the pain or symptoms and maintaining a high vibration (e.g. with thoughts of beauty, love, friendships, etc.). They may also want to visualize themselves as whole and healthy and functioning well. They can continue to practice these exercises at home.

Physical comfort. Keep the person warm, using a blanket, especially if they are wearing light clothing. As the relaxation response progresses, the blood vessels close to the skin will dilate. This causes a cooling of the body, which the client may be too relaxed to notice. If the person is too warm to be covered at the start of a longer session, you might check if their hands are cool after a while and cover the client as the session progresses.

Clients with special physical needs may need attention for positioning. Have extra pillows and bolsters available.

A female patient came to my office for back pain. She was so uncomfortable that it took trying several positions and using many pillows as props for her to tolerate being on the massage table. Half-way through the sequence of back techniques, her pain was not improving and she had to move off the table and sit in a chair to finish. She still had pain when she left my office. I guessed that she went home and took whatever pain meds she had.

Weeks later at a related community support group, another person told me that the same client was claiming to have had a "miracle cure" from me and was pain free. Although back work may take hours or days to shift the energy into balance, I dismissed this report because it was so different from what I observed during and after our session. I thought the person at the support group may have been mistaking me for some other practitioner or even had the wrong client.

About six months after the single treatment, the client came for another appointment, claiming that indeed, she had been pain free for six months and that the pain was returning. It was much less severe than during our first encounter, but she wanted a treatment before it got worse. It seems that the efforts to help her get comfortable contributed to an eventual positive outcome.

Physical pain is one of the most common reasons people seek energy treatments, so it is worth taking the time to help them get comfortable. I remember Janet Mentgen suggesting that, "Once a client is relaxed on the table, your work is half done."

Chronic or long term issues. Clients need to know that chronic or serious conditions with severe energy imbalances may take many sessions for results to be noticed. At times the pain or main symptom may not be relieved, but the client may sleep better or have relief of fatigue. Even if an illness is not cured, the client may find a sense of peace and well-being.

A female client who had diabetes called for Healing Touch in her home. Previously one leg had been amputated below the knee for complications related to diabetes. She had burned the remaining foot with a heat lamp when she was trying to dry a sore at the bottom of her foot to help it heal. Unfortunately, she could not feel the heat due to neuropathy in her foot. At our first meeting there was a small sore (1/4 inch in diameter, perhaps 1/3 inch deep) on the ball of her foot. She was worried that due to poor circulation she would have difficulty healing this wound and would be in danger of losing this leg. I gave her approximately ten treatments. At each treatment I assessed the energy. Each time I felt no energy in her leg until the treatment was completed. During the course of these treatments, the client was also receiving care from physical therapy which included getting fitted for a special shoe that took pressure off her wound. At the time of the fourth session I had a sense that there might be underlying emotional issues. I asked her if there were any unresolved issues that might be creating blocks in her energy field. She revealed issues in relationships with a previous partner and with her son. I suggested that she might try to work with a counselor to help resolve these emotional challenges so that any constricted emotional energy could be available for her healing. She agreed to do so.

When I assessed the field at the start of the tenth session, I noticed for the first time that I could feel the energy in her leg before we started the treatment. Finally, the cumulative effects of the treatments caused the energy balance to "hold." This was a dramatic shift after many weeks. She told me that she noticed the wound had started to heal. Though the news was exciting, it was humbling for me to hear her attribute the healing to her specially designed shoe.

I felt it was somewhat unfortunate that she could not sense the energy of her own field returning, but I thoroughly celebrated her success in healing.

This example shows how long it can take for the energy to re-balance when an issue which has developed over many years (even over a lifetime), and also gives an example of how emotional issues may need to be released for the healing to occur.

CHAPTER 5

ENERGY ASSESSMENT: THE FIELD AND CHAKRAS

Have you ever been able to sense the energy of a room of people, just by being present there? Have you ever sensed the energy or emotions of another person by standing near them? If so, you have some natural ability that otherwise takes discipline and focus to develop.

Assessment of the Energy Field

Before and after energy healing, one can sense the energy in the client's field by gently moving one's hand through the field, a few inches away from the body. When the energy field is balanced and flowing easily the energy will feel even or smooth all over the body. It might feel full, radiant and dynamic. Having terminology to describe the sensations will help ground the assessment process for the healer.

Figure 3

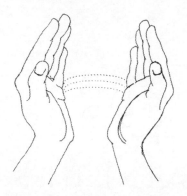

The goal of an energy assessment is to discover where there is congestion or interruption in the smooth flow of energy in the field. To get a sense of how these subtle sensations might feel, hold your hands several feet apart, palms facing each other. Slowly move your palms closer to each other and notice any sensations you feel. Warmth, coolness, static, pressure, resistance, tingling, or hands pulling toward each other are a few of the possible sensations that a person might experience. Each person's field will feel different. Put aside any expectations and try it out! You might be surprised at your ability to feel these and other sensations.

In Healing Touch a pre-treatment assessment will indicate where work is needed. Places in the field that are warmer, cooler, tingly, prickly, or denser than the rest of the field are areas that need to be balanced. Empty places need to be energized. Post-treatment assessments (after the session) show the effectiveness of the treatment.

To assess the energy field of another person:

- Set an intention to accurately sense the energy as needed to give an effective treatment. Hold your hands with palms facing the person's body.
- Sensing the field is a passive, receptive process. Allow the sensations to enter your awareness without attempting to control them.
- Slowly move the hands from head to feet, keeping the hands a few inches from the client's body. Return to any areas you may have missed until all areas are assessed.
- Avoid moving your hands over the same area more than once as it may alter the energy there and be the start of an intervention.

- Observe any sensation you feel in your hands as they move. Particularly notice sensations that feel different from the rest of the field, even if you can't describe them.
- Know also that your other senses may pick up cues about the field. You might experience visual sensations (light, colors), smells, tastes, sounds (static, sparks, chimes, high or low-pitched sounds), or the kinesthetic movement of energy. Your intuition (deep knowing) may bring information to your attention. Your hands might be drawn to an area where specific work is needed. You might notice at times that you can pick up emotions in the client, just by standing near them. However, don't make assumptions based on what you perceive; you can check with the client to see if you are correct.
- Many cues can be taken from the energy. Janet Mentgen reminded practitioners: *Let the energy teach you.*
- Even if you can't directly perceive energy, you *can* give a very good treatment. Have the client tell you where they have pain, injuries, or symptoms and treat those areas for energy imbalances.

Practicing assessments increases one's sensitivity and ability to perceive energy fields. Although the following examples occurred during treatments, they show how perceptions can develop:

I was doing a deep clearing during a Healing Touch treatment for a young woman. She was lying face down. While moving my hands over the back of her legs we both heard what sounded like an electrical spark. She then told me she had metal in her knee.

This next report was given by Susan, a nurse working in an employee healthcare setting:

An employee came to me with a terrible headache. I had her sit down in a chair in the office. From behind her I began to smooth her energy field and then I put my hands on her shoulders. Within maybe five minutes I saw a gray ball of energy the size of a golf ball shoot out of the left side of her head. Immediately she said, "What was that?" She began to move her head and stretch her neck as I told her what I had seen. Her headache was gone. It was really amazing from my point of view.

Assessment of Chakras

The energy of each chakra can be felt by holding a hand over the major chakras. They should feel vibrant and alive, but also be in balance with each other. A pendulum over the chakras will generally move clockwise if the chakra is energized.

Additional Assessment Skills

Visualize the field. There are several ways to begin to learn to see the energy field. One way is to look for an inch or two of distorted light around the client, especially around the head, neck, and shoulders. You can practice holding your hands in front of a plain surface and pulling your fingers apart. You might be able to see strands of energy trailing from your fingers as the hands move away from each other.

You can try using peripheral vision — that is, not looking directly at the field — but perhaps focus on a person's forehead in order to see if you notice the field around the edge of the body. Your eyes might make subtle adjustments for viewing the field. Some describe using *spiritual* vision by closing your eyes and visualizing the field through the *third eye* or brow chakra. Practice looking at everyone you see, as well as animals and plants and trees. Ask for guidance; set your intention to see the field. Be aware that perceiving the energy is a passive, receptive activity. You must *allow* the image to come to your awareness. Straining your eyes or "trying too hard" is not likely to work. For the best results: stay relaxed and practice.

Metaphors. Sometimes a client will describe their symptoms metaphorically. Foot issues might represent not having support or feeling like one does not have *a leg to stand* on. Neck pain could mean that something in the client's life is a *pain in the neck,* or it could signal a fear of *sticking one's neck out.* A person might express feeling pushed or pulled in different directions, which might reflect what is happening to the energy field.

Symbolism in stories may give meaning to a person's journey. After giving treatments to my friend Marsha, I recalled the ancient story of Innana:

Marsha was severely injured in a motor vehicle accident. She had major injuries to her neck, pelvis, ribs, and lungs; with additional problems with sleep, pain, and digestion. Each week the urgency of one symptom surfaced and was treated. The next week another symptom became the focus. It brought to my mind the mythical Sumerian figure of Innana and her descent through the seven gates to the underworld. At each gate she was required to surrender one of her belongings. Although the story does not describe the return of Innana back through the gates and the return of her possessions, as each symptom improved, I felt that Marsha's recovery was like moving through a series of gates. Her functioning improved as each symptom resolved.

In the work of recovering from serious illness or injury, a metaphoric story can offer a focus away from suffering and provide insights that might help bolster one's resolves and strength for healing.

Body Language and Kinesthetics. Some information about the client might be learned by observing posture or facial expressions (happy, sad, worried, stressed, etc). A fidgety client may be anxious. A person in pain often holds his or her hands on the part of their body that hurts, as if naturally directing energy to the painful area. Be aware of the energy of the person as they speak, noticing body language, how fast or slow they are moving and other unspoken cues. Chronic energy imbalances may appear as personality traits.

Using all the senses and intuition with focused awareness will help the healer receive information about the condition of the energy field. This information will be useful in rebalancing the energy field and for giving an optimum energy healing treatment. Whatever information you receive from the client, know that it is still only a portion of their experience. An individual will only share what he or she feels safe sharing from what is accessible in his or her conscious awareness. Even in a lengthy conversation, or if the person is someone you know, you will not learn everything about the client, nor is it necessary. Keep in mind that the energy field is unified and the energy will go where it needs to go. Even just holding a hand and setting an intention could balance the whole field. Many successful healers have used only these simple techniques.

CHAPTER 6

ENERGY TREATMENTS: TECHNIQUES AND RESPONSES

Clearing, Re-balancing and Energizing the Field

It is common to think of healing energy being sent, channeled, or transferred through the energy worker to the client. Another description is that as the energy fields of the healer and client come into contact, there is a transformation taking place. So for example, as the healer's hands move through the field, the congestion in the energy field of the client is not so much swept away as it is transformed or entrained to a higher frequency. Therefore, it is usually not necessary to shake off your hands after clearing energy.

While many techniques are available, using too many techniques in the same session can disrupt the energy field. The simple approaches below can produce dramatic results if used with focus and caring. Janet Mentgen often suggested to those working toward Healing Touch certification that they practice doing a full hour session using only Hands in Motion and Hands Still to understand how simple techniques, when used with awareness, can be quite powerful.

Hands in Motion

Hands in Motion and Hands Still are adapted from Alice Bailey's book called *Esoteric Healing* (1953, 1981).

Figure 4

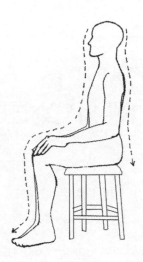

After centering and doing an assessment, hold your palms facing the client's body while gently and slowly sweeping downward and outward, away from the midline. This repeated hand movement clears congested energy of pain, anxiety, or other symptoms and allows the field to re-balance itself. For the whole body, start over the head, neck, and shoulders, repeating downward and outward motion until the energy field feels smooth and clear. Gradually proceed down the front and back of the body and the arms. Then move to the lower body, legs, and feet.

The hand movement may look similar to the assessment. However, the assessment moves over each area only once. Hands in motion might be done over segments of the body, repeating the stokes until each area of the field is clear. Always be observant for how the client is responding. Energy work such as Healing Touch generally relaxes the recipient, but pay attention and stop the treatment if the client becomes restless or uncomfortable. Discomfort is rare, but may be caused by energy moving where it had been previously stagnant or blocked. For example, a limb that has not been used due to pain may experience new sensations as the energy begins to flow through it. Usually the experience is brief and the discomfort is relieved by the end of the session. Be sure to honor any requests to stop the treatment.

Additional points:

- Maintain a heart-centered, caring awareness.
- Although accessing a meditation state is commonly done by closing one's eyes, as practitioner it is best to keep one's eyes open to continually monitor the client's needs and responses.
- The passes are done several inches from the body, at the edge of the etheric field, without touching. Your hand will automatically sense the edge of this field if you don't over-think it.
- The movement downward and outward induces a relaxation response. (Note: Some forms of energy use upward strokes which energize the body. However, for the techniques described here the purpose is to relax the body so it can heal itself.)
- Remember to let the healing energy of the universe flow through you continually. It can energize and balance you as you give a treatment. Then allow the healing energy to flow through your hands. Do not push or force the energy. The client will receive the amount of energy he or she can accept at the time. You might visualize yourself as a clear crystal, with energy flowing through you without any obstruction or judgment. You may need to *get out of the way* if tempted to try to direct the energy. Trust that the energy is going where it needs to go … and you might not know exactly where that is.
- Where the energy is depleted or congested or feels "stuck," it might take many passes to re-balance. The site of the pain, injury, surgery, inflammation, swelling, or other condition may be the main focus. Hands in motion can continue for 5-60 minutes if needed.
- A person who is very sensitive, has severe pain (e.g. burns), has boundary issues, or other issues related to touch may need to have the technique done farther away from the body, possibly several inches or feet.
- Moving too quickly may disrupt the energy field and cause more stress than relaxation.

- Continue Hands in Motion until the energy feels clear, smooth, and vibrant.
- Like many types of treatments, energy healing works better if done as soon as possible after an injury, surgery, or at the onset of symptoms.

In the very early days of Healing Touch, a student reported that her son had injured both legs in a motorcycle accident near their home. While they awaited the ambulance, the family immediately did Healing Touch on the leg that was injured the worst. The student reported that the ER staff was very surprised that the leg with more severe injuries was less swollen and less bruised than the other leg, validating the effect of the energy treatment on that leg.

Hands Still

Hands still can be used before or after Hands in Motion, or as a stand-alone treatment method. Stay centered and let the universal healing energy move through you. Hold your hands on or several inches away from the place where the energy is needed due to pain, injury, or energy congestion. Allow the energy to flow without pushing or forcing it. You can raise your vibration as needed by connecting more deeply with Source, energizing your own chakras, or breathing with awareness.

Hands Still can be done with a focus on the energy centers or with intention to help bones, joints, muscles, organs, the nervous system, the circulatory system, or the immune system. Each type of tissue has a different frequency.

Suggestions for hand positions:

- Position one or both hands comfortably on or near the body where there is pain, a symptom, or an energy disruption.
- Place hands in front and behind the site, or on each side if it is not intrusive to do so. Let the energy flow between your hands
- Energize the joints or energy centers above and below the site being treated.

Balancing and Energizing the Chakras using Hands Still:

- Hold each major chakra with both hands or place one hand in front and one on the corresponding back chakra.

Balancing parts of the body:

- Hold the ankle and hip to treat each leg.
- Hold lower abdomen and heart to treat the torso.
- Hold hand or wrist and shoulder to treat the arm.
- Hold throat or heart and crown to treat the head.
- Use the steps separately for specific symptoms, or in sequence to balance all parts in one session: first each leg, then the torso, next each arm and then the head. (See *Joys' Way,* by Brugh Joy for a description of a complete *Chakra Connection.*)

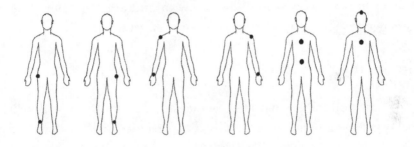

Figure 5

Hold each position until you are aware that the energy has shifted or changed in some way, which means the area might be balanced and energized. The energy may increase and then gradually decrease. Continue until the energy interaction decreases. At other times, you may sense that a warm spot cools or a cold or empty place may start to feel warm and full. You may feel a fullness or pulsations that are the same in each hand. I sometimes sense a rhythm in the interaction of the energy fields, almost like a phrase of music, and feel compelled to hold positions to the end of the phrase. If unable to feel these subtle energy changes, hold each position for one to three minutes. Note: in Reiki and the Brazilian Toe Technique each position is held for at least 3 minutes. I recall the positions even longer may be necessary if the symptoms are severe or long term. I recall that Janet Mentgen recommended holding for another 15 seconds after the energy is balanced in order to stabilize it.

Ending the treatment

When you feel the treatment is complete, re-assess the field and chakras. If the energy field is smooth and even, dynamic, or flowing easily and/or when the energy centers are evenly energized, the treatment is complete. Sometimes clients report when they have relief of pain or other symptoms and feel the treatment is complete. However, continuing until the field is smooth and stable not only allows deeper healing to occur, but also promotes prevention of illness.

Following the treatment, the client may need rest to integrate the changes in the energy field. Allow a few minutes of rest before helping them get up. They may need a nap when they get home.

Grounding the client

Turning off music can help signal the end of the treatment to the client, and begin the grounding process. A client may feel light-headed or day-dreamy after a treatment. They should have time to slowly become alert, so that the effects of the treatment are not undone by sudden awakening. Holding the client's shoulders or feet and offering water to drink can help them return to an alert state. Asking questions which require thoughtful consideration, such as discussing their plans following the session could also help them get grounded. Be sure they are sufficiently alert to get home safely.

For the energy worker, releasing yourself with a sense of loving detachment can help avoid taking on the client's issues. The exchange made for the treatment, such as payment in money or barter of work or goods, can be part of the grounding process, orienting the client and practitioner to the material world. One acupressure worker described that when a payment was made to her after a session, it served as a "protection" and maintained a good boundary between herself and a client's issues.

Client Response

The most common observable effect of energy work is relaxation. Some clients may even fall asleep during a session. It may be that the client's mind goes to the state needed for healing at the time, whether an alert waking state (beta brain waves), a day-dreamy state that can often be accessed just by closing one's eyes (alpha), or a deeper meditation or sleep state (delta, theta, or gamma).

Clients may want to talk about dreams, visions, sensations, memories, or thoughts they had during the session. Avoid interpreting the experiences for them. Encourage them to share what it meant for them and encourage them to allow the meaning to unfold over time.

I remember Janet Mentgen teaching that after a treatment the client may experience a post-hypnotic state in which they are vulnerable to suggestions, until they come to a full alert state. It is an important time to be gentle, to move slowly, and to offer positive feedback. Encourage the client to do some relaxing self care to maintain the effects of the session when they return home.

Asking the client what they noticed during and after the session, especially related to symptoms they reported before the session, can confirm changes that you sensed in the field and shows whether the treatment was effective. Here are some responses of clients who received energy healing:

From my nurse friend Donna after she received a Healing with Colors session:

"It doesn't get any better than this."

Donna also observed that after she gave Healing Touch to her patients they had a different relationship with her. She noticed they made better eye contact and generally seemed appreciative as they recovered from their illnesses.

From a patient at the hospital the evening before surgery, when many would be anxious or tense:

"I have never been so relaxed."

Another nurse reported:

Patients who received Healing Touch were less anxious and seemed more relaxed. They trusted that they would get information as they needed it, rather than push the call button every few minutes.

From Darlene, Midwest USA: The gentle manipulation of craniosacral may or may not be taught as energy work. Darlene clearly interprets this session as an energy treatment.

I am a physician assistant and was working toward Healing Touch certification when I went to try craniosacral work. The office did not have the appearance or ambience of a spa, as some holistic centers. The female practitioner asked some minimal questions and began the treatment. Though I have been practicing Healing Touch and received several other energy treatments, I do not usually have visual experiences during energy work. I had worked in the operating room. However, during this treatment I saw in my mind a room resembling an operating room. I could feel something going on in my body, like a string being pulled. In my mind, I saw two people and could feel etheric sutures being pulled near the area where I had C-sections in the past. When it was over, I felt exhausted and later thought I should have been in a recovery room for spiritual recovery after such an intense treatment.

In the same session, I had a vision of a cottage that I had visited. (In reality the cottage was not in good condition and needed much work. My boyfriend called it a death trap). In the vision I felt the cottage as a place of healing and comfort since the healing opened me to something so deep. I wondered if during that level of healing it was important to be isolated. There was also a kinesthetic experience of cool water running through my body…and a thought of wanting to sell my house and move to the cabin.

After this experience I read in Barbara Brennan's "Hands of Light" book about etheric template surgery performed through the practitioner's hand as if it were an operating room procedure, including the use of etheric instruments.

Occasionally a client's energy field is more chaotic after the session. This may be the result of integration taking place within the field and is not usually cause for concern. Some results unfold over time and may become apparent only after several days. The spine and back, in particular, symbolically may hold the energy of "things we don't want to face" or issues we "turn our backs on." Once after receiving a Healing Touch back session I felt my back pain release exactly 48 hours after the session.

There is a cumulative effect of receiving repeated treatments. The energy field is likely to stay balanced longer with each treatment. This allows the energy healing to go progressively deeper. For example:

When Lauren first started receiving treatments, it took her about twenty minutes just to relax. After a few months it was not unusual for her to go into a deep relaxed state in about five minutes.

Occasionally a client may feel worse before they feel better, as the energy is re-balancing. If an individual has been guarding or protecting an aching part of their body and not using it, that part may have become "frozen." As the energy penetrates into the tissues they may experience some discomfort, but this is usually brief. Some know they can breathe through the pain, just as they would during a deep massage or a medical treatment. If pain occurs during the treatment, let the client know that you can stop anytime, or you may also change to a different technique. Some clients may better tolerate Hands Still if it is done without touching the body; or Hands in Motion when used farther away from the body.

Judy, a friend of mine, had hip replacement surgery in another town. I gave her a Healing Touch treatment when she returned. After the session she told me she had had pain during the treatment, but did not mention it or ask me to stop because she felt the treatment was going deeper into the joint. Her pain was relieved by the end of the session.

Even in a single, brief session, individuals can have a profound experience, such as an opening of their awareness, a sense of initiation, or an alchemical process. Therefore, treatments are often a welcoming of the client into a new state of being. These same initiatory experiences might also take place in a Healing Touch class. Students who are expecting to learn techniques and theory, may step into their personal transformation. At times the energy can feel like an overload. It may bring into focus emotions or memories that the person had been attempting to bury. The instructor or practitioner cannot control these events, but can be supportive and stay grounded while helping clients to stay grounded as well.

At the end of one Level 1 Healing Touch class, several women were tearful when talking about what they had gotten out of the class. One was able to articulate that she had been able to make contact with a part of herself that was cut off for many years. Another felt a sense of letting go and forgiveness long after having been molested. Another spoke of how the class helped her to finally feel safe and comforted.

Babies and very young children, as well as the elderly may be more sensitive to energy than others. They might need brief treatments. Restlessness might be a sign that they have had enough. For all clients, it is good for the healer to keep his or her eyes open and be attentive to the client's response. Be prepared to stop or change your technique if necessary.

An elderly woman hospitalized for knee surgery received a Healing Touch treatment from me and another practitioner friend, Darcy. After fifteen minutes of relaxation she became restless. We ended the session, knowing it was enough for her at the time.

It is good practice to let go of the outcomes, since results may be different than what was expected. For example, *one client wanted energy healing for an ear infection and later reported she was not craving cigarettes.*

Healing is a complex process, with many individual differences. The client may not always perceive the results because the work being done may relate to a deeper psychological or spiritual need on a different level of awareness. Some clients request pain relief but may instead, or in addition, feel more peaceful or whole.

One client who had fibromyalgia and trauma issues received a Healing Touch treatment from me. She had had previous energy treatments with acupressure so I did some deeper work. After the treatment, she seemed in a hurry to leave and dashed out of my office without much time for getting grounded. A third party later reported that the client felt worse physically after the session. However, by the time I actually saw the client, she told me that she did have some emotions release and felt better in the end.

It seems in this case the work may have stirred up issues energetically on the physical level, although some healing occurred at the emotional level. This example also shows that the energy process may need time to integrate before it has the desired effect.

A younger woman became agitated during a session while receiving some deeper work using Barbara Brennan's techniques. She thought the music was too stimulating. I intuitively sensed it was the intensity of the technique. I changed the music and continued with a less intensive technique and the session proceeded without difficulty.

Energy work can also clear away superficial defenses that we use unconsciously to protect ourselves from emotional pain. There have been several instances where a client felt anger or grief during or after a session. This does not mean that energy work caused the emotion, but that it brought an issue into focus, possibly after clearing more superficial issues.

Client responses are as varied as presenting symptoms. A change in the symptoms is a sign the energy is moving and the person's energy field is shifting to a state of energetic balance, which could happen quickly or over time. Always observe the client for how they are tolerating the treatment. It might be necessary to alter an approach by using hands off the body instead of hands on or using a different technique, or shortening the session – to help a client be more comfortable.

Work in Groups

Whether in the hospital or at home, friends and family can be guided to help give in a treatment. Providing the comfort of a healing treatment is usually a welcome change from sitting worrying about their loved one. At the hospital I often ask visitors or staff if they would like to help with the treatment.

One woman requested Healing Touch in the hospital before surgery. Her husband was with her and I invited him to help with the treatment. I gave him the briefest explanation, instructing him about where to put his hands so that we could balance the energy field before surgery. I suggested that he send love through his hands or hold love in his heart. The patient smiled and was moved by this treatment. I noticed a tear in her eye.

Another woman was in the infusion room at the hospital receiving chemotherapy, and had four friends visiting. With simple instructions from me, they put their hands on her and gave a wonderful caring Healing Touch treatment. The looks on the faces of patient and visitors showed that a profound bonding experience was shared.

A woman was visited by her husband and two daughters after surgery. We gave the patient a treatment together. It was inspiring to see how some people are willing to try something they have never seen before to help a loved one. They were rewarded by seeing their mom/wife relaxed and in less pain.

Keeping Notes

You may want to keep notes related to what the client needed, the assessment, what you did, and the results. Be sure to maintain confidentiality for all records, keeping them stored in a safe place, preferably one that is locked.

The notes can help recall information about a client you have not seen for several weeks or months. Documentation can also reveal patterns in the energy field, which techniques were most helpful, and the progress toward healing.

Rites of Passage

Most students have a positive experience from energy healing classes, particularly Healing Touch, in which there is extensive training and certification of instructors. Several things occur in classes that promote transformation, at times of an unexpected magnitude. For one, doing energy work in a group tends to magnify the experience which can create greater results and a more intense experience than a one-to-one treatment outside of the classroom. Secondly, the number of treatments given and received during training also has a cumulative and multiplied effect. Janet Mentgen, the founder of Healing Touch, understood a great deal about energy and designed the standardized curriculum so that the techniques occur in a specific sequence to be effectively presented in class. For those who are ready, this structure provides a passage into one's own deeper being, which may be experienced as an initiation at each level. Others who are exploring Healing Touch to get a sense of what it is about tend to have a more superficial experience in a caring environment, learning techniques that can help themselves and others. A few others leave the class untouched by the energy, or even a bit overwhelmed.

Healing Crisis

A healing crisis is a reaction that can occur as a result of bodywork. In massage therapy it is described as the result of stored toxins being released into the system, creating a temporary state of discomfort that can last hours or even days. While a similar experience might cause some people to think that the energy work made them worse, it is more often a sign that the treatment has been effective. Though it is rare, a *healing crisis* during or after energy work might be a physical, emotional, mental, or spiritual experience.

The student below experienced the death of a close relative sometime before a Healing Touch training class occurred, and had the memory of the person come back to her during the class. She shared this experience:

I first heard about energy healing from a nurse who took care of me and my baby 15 years ago at a hospital. It took 13 years until I was able to find a class that was offered and I eagerly jumped at the opportunity. It was a weekend class and was absolutely fascinating. We had somewhere around 15 classmates and we had discussions and practice on each other. Every other classmate eventually acknowledged "feeling" the energy from others when they worked on them, and sometimes when they were being worked on. I was the only one who never felt anything at all. However, I was still enthusiastic and eager to meet together as a group to practice later on, and to volunteer at the hospital to work on patients before and after surgery as requested by certain doctors. I was excited about these opportunities, about eventually "getting it" and feeling the energy, and about being able to use this new gift.

However, the day after class ended I woke up plunged in a horribly deep, awful, heavy depression. It was mostly physical I would say, but it was so awful that the only thing I could make myself do was to get up, get my kids breakfast, see them to the bus stop, and go back to lie on the couch the rest of the day, wrapped tightly in a quilt or blanket, for the next week and a half. At the end of the day I would drag myself back up to make dinner for my family. I could not even make myself use the Bach Flower Remedies, for which I am a practitioner.

The following Sunday, which was six days into it, I got myself to church as usual. The routine, the association, and the usual Sunday jobs I had began to pull me out of it a little bit. This started me being able to help myself. The whole depression thing ended 10 days after it started.

This ten day depressive episode is an example of a healing crisis that may have been triggered by her experience of being in the intensive energy of a class. Perhaps her inability to not feel the energy was part of a defense. The energy experienced in class may have broken through that defense and brought emotions to the surface. While further sessions of clearing and balancing may have helped and were offered, she declined. Others may experience something similar, though usually much less dramatic. These episodes are not always easily explained, since life is complex and there are many contributing factors to our experiences.

Referrals

While the most common response to energy work is a relaxed sense of peace and well-being, energy work can bring up many issues and may result in tears, sobbing, laughter, or a need to talk. Aware listening skills are important, but avoid giving advice or counseling if you are not a counselor. Think about being a witness to what the client is experiencing, or *holding the light*, that is, holding a positive intention for them. Energy workers must be clear about their own skills for handling concerns that arise beyond the scope of their practice, training, or abilities and know when it is appropriate to refer a client to another professional. Some clients need additional medical help, counseling, massage, or other professional evaluation and treatment.

Collaboration

Collaborative work also is an interesting option. *I gave a couple of Healing Touch sessions to a client with his therapist present. The therapist was able to help him move out of a stuck place emotionally, while I could fully attend to the energy treatment to free the congested emotional energy. In this way, he received the benefit of both approaches and was able to process some issues more quickly and effectively.*

Effects on Medication

Energy healing can have an effect on medications, usually potentiating them, that is, making them have a greater effect. Clients may notice that they need to use less pain medication; however, clients must always work with their prescribing caregiver if they wish to change medication doses. For example, one diabetic client reported needing less insulin while receiving weekly energy treatments.

How Often to Give Treatments

The frequency of treatments may be dictated by time available, but treatments are most beneficial if a client receives energy healing as often as is necessary to maintain balance. For example, a client who just had surgery and has a depleted field may need a treatment once or twice a day until they can hold a balance for longer. Then treatments can be given every two or three days and progress as the energy field stabilizes. For long term issues, many treatments may be needed. Most people tend to schedule routine sessions on a weekly basis so it is easier to keep track of the appointments. After acute issues are resolved, some clients continue to receive energy healing for maintenance.

Lauren received Healing Touch for several years. Initially she received treatments for a fracture of the humerus (upper arm) that was not healing well, as well as a hip replacement. Once these areas were healed, she continued to have treatments whenever her schedule would permit. She felt the maintenance treatments help her to "re-set" her energy and stay balanced during her stressful work days.

Effective energy treatments can be given, even with the simple techniques described in this chapter. Working in another person's energy field is a complex interaction with the vibrations of body, mind, and spirit. An energy worker needs to keep their own energy field open, stay focused and centered, and be always aware of the client's response. The next chapter on Ethics, describes respecting boundaries to protect client and healer in maintaining a healing relationship for optimal results.

CHAPTER 7

ETHICS: GUIDELINES FOR
A NEW PARADIGM

Guidelines for Conduct

Ethics are rules that govern acceptable behavior between people. In general ethical behavior involves being accountable, using good judgment, abiding by laws and respecting the rules of one's profession. In providing a health-related service, workers are encouraged to follow the guideline, "Above all else do no harm". This phrase is from the Hippocratic Oath taken by nurses and doctors. It provides a powerful reminder for energy workers to not knowingly do anything that will cause harm to clients.

Janet Mentgen would sometimes reflect on the two types of errors committed in nursing. The first type was an error of commission, which is when something is done incorrectly. The second type was an error of omission, when a nurse failed to do something needed for the care of the patient. If nurses knew about Healing Touch and did not use it when they knew it would help a patient, Janet wondered, "Were they committing an error of omission?"

Energy Healing that is non-invasive is not likely to have negative side-effects. However, as more people aspire to doing healing work, new situations arise that bring to light the need for guidelines to protect both the giver and receiver of energy work. Some holistic modalities seem simple and the mechanics of some techniques can be learned in an evening class or by reading a book. The actual interactions of care are more complicated and better learned with professional training, mentoring, or supervised experience.

When individuals are employed in organizations, behavior is guided by rules which provide protection during interactions and there is supervision. However, the work of energy healing may be the first experience some people will have in the role as an independent worker giving a treatment to a private client outside the sheltered structure of a class or organization. For this reason it is important to consider what is ethical when giving energy healing treatments.

Touch is a deeply personal experience. Ethical behavior demands that an individual is asked before being touched. Survivors of trauma and many types of abuse are especially aware of boundary issues and may prefer non-contact treatments. It is also important to research the laws regarding touch in your state. Some states have laws about who is licensed to do any work that involves touching another person. A number of states now have Health Freedom laws that allow non-licensed practitioners to give treatments that are not invasive or medical treatments.

When in a role of helping someone, energy workers might be perceived as having certain skills and power. This is called *The White Coat Effect*. This effect results in the client making the assumption that the care provider is knowledgeable and responsible, and has certain innate authority. Because of this effect, it is important to practice only the skills that you are trained and authorized to use. There are strict laws about practicing medicine without a license. Be sure to decline requests for skilled care that is beyond your training and credentials, even if the client encourages you in some way. Refer clients to other health professionals when needed. Avoid giving advice in integrative methods without training and refer clients to nutritionists, homeopaths, herbologists, or other licensed and trained professionals if needed. Suggest they do their own research to learn about additional treatments beyond what you are qualified to offer. In holistic practice there is an emphasis on encouraging clients to make conscious choices about their health so that they can be a partner in their care. We also need to respect those choices even if we don't agree with them.

A female patient with a young daughter decided to stop chemotherapy for cancer. Her decision was very difficult for the nurses going to her home to give Healing Touch treatments. Some believed that chemotherapy would give her some chance of longer survival to be with her young daughter. Even worse, the patient was unable to quit smoking. The nurses needed to set aside their own beliefs about chemo and their knowledge about healthy lifestyle choices in order to continue providing care. The patient did continue to receive Healing Touch until her death.

A young woman with ovarian cysts came to my office. Her goal was to shrink the cysts. She knew the size of the cysts because of an ultrasound test. She came in for four Saturday morning treatments. She also agreed that she would do some visualization of the cysts shrinking when she was at home. At each Saturday morning appointment she smelled of alcohol, which was still leaving her system from the night before. At the fourth session I talked to her again about self care. I suggested that decreasing her intake of alcohol might improve her body's ability to heal the cysts, since the body had to do the added work of detoxing the alcohol. Her non-response gave the impression that she was not interested in giving up drinking. Then she told me the most recent ultrasound showed that the cysts were significantly smaller and that she was satisfied with the treatments. She made no additional appointments. I never saw her again.

Some energy workers have clients sign an informed consent before receiving a treatment. The consent may include the credentials of the practitioner, a definition of the modality and what the patient can expect, how to report a grievance, etc. It may not be necessary to have a client sign a written informed consent document. However, be sure that clients know your name, credentials, and level of training for doing energy work. They should understand the energy treatment procedure they are to receive and have an idea of what to expect. They should also be informed of the limitations of the treatment, such as in a case where perhaps the condition may not be curable. Explanations about energy healing are best given in generalities rather than specifics so as to avoid making promises, agreements, or guarantees that such treatments can cure cancer or other health challenges.

While some individuals will be strongly attracted to energy work and Healing Touch classes or treatment, not all people need, want or can accept energy work. Avoid trying to convince people about the benefits of energy healing and pay attention to subtle cues when someone might be politely and gently declining your services. Some people have strict religious beliefs or personal preferences that are to be respected.

I passed by a hospital room where a female patient was coughing and having mild respiratory distress. I offered her Healing Touch, but she replied, "No, thanks. I'm a prayer person."

Although prayers and energy healing work well together for most people, I respected her personal way of declining and did not try to convince her.

Ethics also extend to the sphere of information collecting. Personal information that someone reveals during an energy treatment should be kept confidential. If anything from a session is put in writing, it should be locked in a secure place.

Ethical practice includes not discriminating against anyone because of age, race, culture, gender, beliefs, or lifestyle issues. Some types of energy healing, such as Healing Touch, have Standards for Practice or a Code of Ethics that are guidelines for ethical behavior.

Some practitioners may charge money or have some means of exchange or barter for a treatment, particularly if energy work is done as part of an established profession, such as massage. The energy worker should have a certain amount of proficiency before charging a fee. Rates are typically comparable to massage therapy.

Professional Relationships/ Good Boundaries

Energy work such as Healing Touch is done either without physical contact, or with gentle, non-sexual light touch. It is not massage.

Providing energy treatments with a caring, heart-centered attitude allows clients to feel safe. Even energy work done without touching can create a sense of intimacy. Keeping good boundaries starts with explaining clearly what will happen in a session and staying on track with those expectations. When roles are understood and boundaries respected, it allows both client and energy worker to access deeper parts of themselves emotionally and spiritually and can make the treatment more effective. However, poor boundaries create vulnerability. Understanding some of the dynamics of a therapeutic relationship can help the energy worker steer clear of problems.

Transference and counter-transference are psychotherapy terms used to describe aspects of the practitioner-client relationship that can be developed, challenged, and used for a therapeutic purpose. Although energy healing is not psychotherapy, the aspects of caring and focused attention on the client's issues may provoke similar dynamics. Transference relates to the feelings a client has about the therapist, usually based on unconscious projections the client makes that relate to a parent. Counter-transference describes the reaction the therapist has to the client, and is the result of unfulfilled needs or other unconscious agendas on the part of the therapist. The feelings in either direction can be positive or negative and easily misinterpreted by vulnerable clients or practitioners. When a client or therapist falls in love or begins to have unexplained resentments toward the other, it is likely that transference or counter-transference is the cause. Energy workers have the responsibility to maintain boundaries and receive consultation as needed in order to work through transference or counter-transference.

Using good listening skills in energy work allows the client to share experiences and emotions. Although a client may share much personal information and use the energy healing session to "vent," it is not a psychotherapy or counseling session. An energy healing worker should not take on the role of counselor if he or she is not a trained counselor. Refer clients to counseling if they need more help than you are qualified or licensed to give.

Choosing Clients

The best clients for energy healing are those who are able and willing to give consent on their own, and who can give feedback openly e.g. about how the treatment is going. Individuals who are paranoid, psychotic, unable to understand, out of touch with reality, impaired by substance abuse, or who may misinterpret the intent of the treatment are not good candidates.

One time a woman called to ask about taking a class. She belonged to a fundamentalist religion and was not sure if Healing Touch would be approved by her church. She asked if I would talk to her minister to find out if it was okay for her to take a class. Her approach revealed enough to show me that an energy class was not for her. I declined to contact her minister and she did not pursue taking the class.

When working at an outpatient center for treating the chronically mentally ill, I would give occasional Healing Touch demonstrations to staff and higher functioning clients. At one presentation, a patient who was very psychotic wandered into the group in the large meeting room and watched me demonstrating Hands in Motion as I moved my hands around an individual's head. "I know what you are doing," the visitor said. "You are taking your psyche and putting it into HER psyche."

This, of course, was a dramatic misinterpretation on the part of the patient. Other psychiatric patients may unconsciously incorporate similar misunderstandings into their delusions. If a patient sees you as a witch or alien (which is not unusual in the world of psychiatry) it could be frightening to them as well as you. It would be best to not offer energy healing in questionable situations such as these.

Some healers believe that energy workers should never work on their own family or friends. However, in many cases, excellent treatments have been provided by friends or family members. It is important to recognize one's vulnerabilities and assess whether one can give a treatment without emotional interference of resentments, strained expectations, manipulations, and other unhealthy dynamics that sometimes occur unconsciously in familial relationships.

Complicated dynamics of dual relationships can also occur when giving treatments to friends or co-workers. Unspoken agendas and role confusion can sometimes affect the treatment or awkwardly reshape a continuing relationship. For example, if a co-worker shares information about their illness or relationship struggles in the safety of a session, they may feel self-conscious later in the workplace. The energy worker might feel burdened by this unexpected revelation as well. In any case, be sure to keep the boundaries clear between the session and the other interactions you may have with a client.

When first learning energy healing techniques, it is common for the student to enthusiastically offer sessions to as many people as possible, since practice is important. However, discerning which individuals are appropriate candidates will ensure mutual satisfaction for client and healer.

Liability

Although energy work is gentle and subtle and unlikely to cause harm, there are liability issues that can arise. Misrepresenting your skills, intentions, and credentials, could be cause for litigation. Making promises, such as being able to cure a condition could lead to breaking a trust with the client or with the public and be a liability. For those who set up a business practice, there are legal city and state procedures to follow.

Service

Whether or not fees are involved, giving energy treatments, including distance healing, is providing a service. While some healers charge a fee for service, others may opt to provide free treatments to those unable to pay, or for family members.

In her book *Born to Serve: The Evolution of the Soul Through Service,* Susan Trout, PhD, describes several levels of service. The lowest level is one in which an individual does service without any specific commitment related to the service, but merely because it is an expectation of a group in which they are a member. The levels progressively relate to service that is more deliberate and selfless. She discusses the highest level of service as one in which the giver of the service does not know who is the receiver and the one receiving does not know the sender or even that a service is being done. Holding energy for resolution of world conflicts or maintaining a high vibration in general could be considered this level of service.

Rachel Naomi Remen had this to say on the topic of service: "Helping, fixing, and serving represent three different ways of seeing life. When you help, you see life as weak. When you fix, you see life as broken. When you serve, you see life as whole. Fixing and helping may be the work of the ego, and service the work of the soul."

CHAPTER 8

SELF CARE FOR ENERGY WORKERS AND CLIENTS

Lifestyle Enhancement

Energy workers who practice self care will improve the quality of their work and have a better understanding of the challenges involved in helping clients make changes in behavior and attitude. Self care is important because it helps the practitioner maintain a balanced energy field. Being as healthy and rested as possible will help the energy worker to be present and focused on the client's needs. Clients are also encouraged to work on self care to promote their own healing. Self care is good for everyone.

In the realm of holistic care there are many lifestyle enhancement approaches a person can take to promote health and healing. Although some approaches may seem more directed toward body, mind, or spirit and are organized in that manner in the next section, holistic care affects the whole person. For example, a breathing exercise increases the amount of oxygen brought to the cells and calms the mind and emotions. As a form of meditation, it connects a person to spirit. Therefore a breathing exercise can be viewed as a practice that helps body, mind, and spirit.

All of the activities listed in this section hold the possibility of raising your vibration or keeping your vibration high to promote health of body, mind, and spirit. Additionally, a positive attitude creates a higher vibration than one based on fear, worry, or negative expectations.

Pay attention to whether a self care activity is working. If a plan is not getting expected or desired results in a reasonable time, reevaluate whether another choice is needed.

The topic of change can evoke mixed reactions for those of us who see ourselves as creatures of habit. Both in psychiatric nursing and holistic health, behavior change is a focus for many patients and clients. The Stages of Change – pre-contemplation, contemplation, action, maintenance, and relapse – provide a means of assessing the type of information and support individuals need at specific times in their process. Correct interventions given at the appropriate times are more likely to be successful. Knowing that change is a process with defined stages can be helpful.

Energy Healing for Self Care

There is a natural reflex to put one's hand on the pain when a body part is injured or has a symptom. It seems to be part of the inner wisdom of a human being. Learning energy healing could be thought of as an extension of that natural reflex, or accessing our inner wisdom to help ourselves and each other.

Cleansing one's own energy field can also be done by washing hands, taking a shower, or soaking in a bath with eight ounces of baking soda. Many of the self care approaches listed below will help balance the energy field as well.

Hands in Motion can be used on oneself, wherever the hands can reach. Use Hands Still by placing your hand on or near the area that needs energy and set an intention to have the energy penetrate through the body to that area. Trust that the energy will go where it is needed. Balancing major and minor chakras can be done on one's own legs, arms, torso, and head. Another way to work on yourself is to imagine that someone else is giving you a treatment, especially for the areas that you cannot reach. You can also visualize golden light balancing and healing the area in need.

Physical Self care

Breathing. One of the simplest self care exercises involves paying attention to each breath without counting or breathing in any particular way. Position your body so that your back is straight but not rigid, while lying on the floor or sitting. Even a few moments of placing attention on the breath will have a relaxing effect. Increase the length of time as you are able. Focused breathing can be used to ease a tense moment at work, reduce addictive cravings, or raise vibrations for more meaningful personal interactions.

Movement such as stretching, yoga, or aerobic exercise releases tension and stiffness and reminds the mind and body about good posture and what it means to truly feel well. Exercise increases circulation which helps the functioning of all parts of the body. Research is revealing the importance of exercise, not just for heart health, but also to preserve brain functioning (Daniel Amen, MD on PBS TV).

Diversion and Rest. Taking breaks from sitting, computer time, or strenuous work will refresh your mind and body and prevent injury from repetitive activity. The brain can function better when it has brief intervals of diversion. When one is tired from doing the same activities or types of work diversion is needed. If one is tired from doing different types of activity then rest is needed.

Sleep. Two or three decades ago, eight hours of sleep was an accepted norm for many people. Now there are huge numbers of people who survive on much less sleep because of stress, anxiety, pain, sleep apnea, unreasonable work responsibilities, homelessness, safety issues, poor social situations, or other issues. The body needs sleep to repair itself and maintain health. There is no substitute. Lack of sleep can result in psychosis, depression, inability to think or make good decisions, lowered frustration tolerance, hostility, weight gain, and many other problems. Relaxation, guided imagery tapes, energy work, meditation, aromatherapy, certain herbs or dietary supplements, and avoiding stimulants such as caffeine can improve sleep. If not, consider getting additional help.

Water. For some people the simplest improvement in physical health might be made by drinking more water. The current way of life for many involves exposures to pollution in the air, toxins in water and the environment, additives in foods, and exposure to chemicals and infectious organisms. Drinking clean water in adequate amounts can help the liver and the kidneys filter out some of these substances and prevent illness. Water is needed by all cells in the body, including the neurons of the brain. One study showed that 37% of Americans had a thirst mechanism so weak that they mistake thirst for hunger. Research at the University of Washington showed that one glass of water shut down midnight hunger pangs for almost 100% of the dieters in one study. Even a 2% drop in body water can trigger fuzzy short term memory, trouble with basic math and difficulty focusing on the computer screen or a printed page. Some research showed that drinking 8-10 glasses of water per day could ease back and joint pain. It is however possible to drink too much water, resulting in yet other physical problems, including water intoxication, so keep it within reasonable limits.

Nutrition. The USDA's most recent suggestion for balanced food groups shows a plate divided into four sections (see choosemyplate.gov). The vegetable and grain sections are slightly larger than the protein and fruit sections and there is a serving of dairy on the side.

Avoiding preservatives, additives, pesticides, and known allergens can go a long way to improving health and decreasing inflammation. Organic foods are becoming more available in grocery stores and are an excellent option as well.

When you are sensitive to the energy field, you will be more aware of which foods are needed for you to function at your best. Healthy foods have a high vibration and keep the body's vibration high. Processed foods have a lower vibration which depletes a person's energy field. Trusting and following intuition or inner wisdom might lead to more success than following diets marketed for profit or eating plans that might not be for your specific body type.

Clearing space. In one's living and work spaces, the "stuff" collected there and how it is arranged – will affect a person's energy field. One teacher suggested that *one's closets reflect the condition of one's mind.* Feng Shui provides principles that help the flow of energy in a space. Often the first guideline is to get rid of clutter. Janet Mentgen taught that material possessions hold energy. If those belongings are from dysfunctional relationships, bad decisions, or failures, then a person may be inadvertently surrounded with energy that is blocking a more positive personal agenda.

A while back, I was going through my bookshelves to clear out books I was no longer using. I had ordered sets of EFT videos around the same time. When the tapes arrived, they took up the exact amount of space that I had just cleared on the shelf. For me it was a good metaphor for making space for the new things I was inviting into my life.

Relaxation. Using any method of relaxation provides the benefits of slowing the heart rate and decreasing blood pressure — both of which lower stress on the body's organs. Relaxation also decreases muscle tension and enables the body to have more energy, better sleep, improved immunity, less pain, increased concentration, better problem solving ability and even emotional stability.

Emotional and Mental Self Care

The mind is a powerful force in healing, and provides us with a great benefit if our thoughts and attitudes are empowering. Emotions relate to feelings, whereas mental processes relate to our thoughts and attitudes.

Positive stress is a motivator nudging us to take action for the benefit of ourselves or others. However, too much stress or the wrong kind of stress is disruptive and harmful, rendering a person less functional. While stress is generally felt as an emotional or mental experience causing poor attitude, failure of decision-making abilities, and decreased self-esteem, prolonged stress can have a serious effect on all systems of the body. The effect is cyclical: stress causes illness or makes it worse; illness causes more stress. Adding one or more of the following holistic self help activities can make the difference between surviving or coping with life or actually thriving while achieving balance and reaching healthy goals.

Journal writing is a self help tool for expressing emotions on paper and processing ideas or conflicts. Journaling also helps one to expand spiritually. A suggestion for those new at journal writing is to write about how you are doing physically, emotionally, mentally and spiritually (PEMS), and addressing any goals related to those areas. Making these notes regularly such as daily, weekly or monthly, can help clarify your experiences and show your progress. Journaling can also point out places where you might be stuck (when the same thing is written each month), and when you need to put more attention on an issue or to reach out for help.

Writing unsent letters is a journal exercise that can be used to release old conflicts with a person. If the person is no longer available, or if it would be harmful to confront them, writing an unsent letter can help release anger, grief or other feelings without needless humiliation or placing oneself in danger.

Journaling in a dialogue format can be used to get in touch with the emotional cause of a symptom, by having a conversation with the body part, an illness, or even an addiction. Ask what that symptom is trying to tell you. Then write a response from that aspect of yourself (as if the symptom is speaking through you and to you). The wise mind has the information to answer questions about causes and solutions for one's problems. This dialogue technique creates a framework for accessing that wisdom.

Writing about dreams, or spiritual or intuitive experiences — including coincidences, insights, guidance, healing experiences, or experiences of perceiving energy — can help to expand spiritual awareness. Writing a list of things for which a person is grateful often reverses a negative attitude and helps to raise one's vibration.

A number of years ago I read Diane Wardell's book *White Shadow*, in which she described her own journaling process and that of Janet Mentgen. I was inspired to journal daily for a few weeks, specifically about the healing treatments I was giving. Immediately I began to have experiences with clients that were beyond the usual treatment for pain and stress that were more typical in my practice at the time. I believe that the journaling process helped me to be sufficiently grounded for these events to occur. Here is one example:

I had sent a letter to psychotherapists and counselors explaining the benefits of Healing Touch and how it might help their clients release emotions or behavior patterns that are "stuck." One of the therapists who responded was a friend of mine. The client she referred was a young woman who had given birth to a stillborn baby one month prior. The therapist reported that the client was doing well, but she thought that energy healing might offer something additional. The client agreed.

During the treatment I intuitively felt the baby's energy still present. I was reluctant to share that with the client. I did not want to stir up emotions for her. Yet, as the client sat up, she immediately asked, "What did you feel?"

I acknowledged that I did feel the energy of the baby. The client quickly shared that she felt the baby as well, and then suddenly she felt the baby's energy release. She knew that she herself had already let go of the baby, but felt the baby's spirit had not let go until this session. She felt a tremendous release during this experience and was grateful for being able to heal at another level.

The Emotional Freedom Technique (EFT) is a self care technique that consists of tapping acupuncture meridians to rebalance the energy field. The major meridians generally begin at the finger tips and toes and end in major organs. Acupuncture uses needles to stimulate the meridians to release chemicals into the organs to balance the energy of the body and have a healing effect. EFT uses tapping instead of needles. Anyone can learn EFT. Tutorials, books and newsletters are readily available on the internet (See Gary Craig, Carol Look, Nick Ortner and others). This remarkable technique is easy to use and can be done anywhere and anytime. EFT is a good approach for managing stress, problem solving, and making wise choices. Its greatest benefit may be in the deeper applications of clearing old emotions and memories from past experiences which still influence our daily choices.

When I first learned EFT I was having low levels of anxiety. I tried tapping on releasing the anxiety for fifteen minutes every morning and evening for four days. I then had no anxiety for three months.

One woman used EFT after participating in a demonstration I gave. The next day she told me that she used it for asthma and did not need her extra inhaler.

I woke up with some neck pain that I had been having, plus the feeling that my neck was out of alignment. I did EFT on the alignment issue for a few minutes. Some of the pain remained, but I no longer felt out of alignment.

EFT can be used for pain relief, changing behavior and attitudes, releasing addictions and unhealthy cravings, helping to heal many physical symptoms, improving concentration, and achieving goals.

Meditation is a time-honored self care practice that uses an inward focus to quiet the mind. Meditation might be described as *releasing each thought as it comes into awareness.* There are many types of meditation. The breathing exercise described earlier (placing attention on each breath) is a good beginning meditation. Repeating a *mantra* or a calming word or phrase such as *Peace* or *I am in the Light* is the basis for several types of meditation. Focusing on an intention for the healing of self or others could also be useful.

Visualizing a situation as you would like it to be might help the mind to bring that situation into reality. This could be used to heal oneself, heal another person, or even to help a situation. The use of **imagery** is an expanded type of visualization whereby other senses, in addition to vision, are brought into play in order to imagine a possibility. A *mini-vacation* is a stress management technique where one imagines the perfect vacation that is both enjoyable and stress free. Some people benefit a great deal from this brief experience, where luggage does not get lost, no one gets sick, the weather is perfect, and flights are not delayed.

Mindfulness is a practice in which one is non-judgmental and fully aware of the reality in the present moment. This can lead to calmness in one's daily life.

Affirmations are positive statements voiced in the present tense for the purpose of achieving goals and self empowerment. A few examples include: I am getting healthier each day; I can heal this illness; I am attracting positive healthy people into my life.

Perhaps the best affirmation I have ever heard came from my friend Rebecca: I am a brilliant reflection of the vibrant energies of the universe.

Biofeedback has helped many people to achieve relaxation. The feedback is in the form or audio or visual cues that change as one relaxes. For example, a sound feedback might be a high pitched tone that lowers as one's muscle tension relaxes. Biofeedback helps people to learn that they can actually control impact of stress on the body. One computer program called *Journey Through the Wild Divine* is a self help approach that monitors physiological changes through the use of a small finger electrode. As relaxation increases the user is able to successfully complete tasks on the visual screen as part of a game. In contrast to violent computer games, this journey features aesthetic displays and peaceful landscapes, all while guiding a person to attain deeper levels of relaxation.

Psychotherapy/counseling. Holistic self care can work on nearly everything. The important thing is to notice whether it is working or not. Sometimes it is beneficial or necessary to get help (or an outside perspective) from therapists or counselors. Negotiate clear goals with your therapist and evaluate the goals together regularly.

Social Support. As humans, social support provides a necessary safety net. Caring for others and being cared for by others helps to keep each person whole. Whether the support is from family, friends, support groups, Twelve Step work, or other relationships, nurturing these connections contributes to overall health.

There are many **additional energy approaches** that can be part of a self care practice. Herbs, crystals, homeopathy, and healing sounds are other examples of approaches that use the effect of vibrations to create healing. Humor, laughter, dance, pets, music, and letting go are also beneficial. Personalized rituals can be a way of marking a choice such as starting an exercise program, or celebrating a success, like giving up an addiction. Personalizing the ritual means you can create a new, healthy way to celebrate. The ritual could be a private event that includes a walk in nature, a hot bath, a spa day. A group activity might involve playing music, a talking circle, a healthy food potluck dinner, or a hike.

The Environment

Experiencing the environment as part of ourselves is most likely how humans are meant to exist. The more we can protect and heal the environment the better our chance of having clear air, safe water, and less toxins, which will make it easier to maintain our own health. Buying only sustainably produced items when possible can give a sense of connection to a bigger world. Such items are manufactured with both the Earth and the worker who made them in mind. Re-using, recycling, and avoiding use of fossil fuels when possible are simple steps to help global problems. The avoidance of buying unnecessary goods also goes a long way in helping the Earth.

Spiritual Balance

Maintaining spiritual balance enriches a holistic lifestyle, and can be especially important for holistic energy workers. Since individuals define spirituality for themselves, spiritual expression can take different forms. Having meaning and purpose is one way of describing spirituality. Whether we connect with the forces greater than ourselves through prayer, meditation, gardening or helping others is a personal matter. Art, music, song and chanting can help a person connect to his or her deeper self. Being outdoors in fresh air and natural beauty can reduce stress and help us remember our connection to earth and spirit. For many people being in nature helps connect with the Source.

Forgiveness of Self and Others. Forgiveness never means that the harm someone has done to you was okay. It means letting go of the power that the experience has over you. You are doing this for yourself when you are ready, so you can be your own true self. You're not doing it for the perpetrator. Forgive everything. It really isn't that hard. Call your spirit back from being stuck in resentments. And if you are able, forgive things before they happen.

Twelve Step Wisdom. Twelve Step programs such as Alcoholics Anonymous (AA), Over-eaters Anonymous (OA), and others offer recovery of body, mind, and spirit for those who suffer with addictions. As a cognitive and behavioral approach these programs promote "right action" such as abstaining from harmful behavior. Working the steps offers a framework for spiritual self-improvement that includes making amends, and connecting to a Higher Power.

The Hero's Journey. The commitment to become active in one's own healing process may demand discipline or even lead to an unexpected spiritual or emotional life journey. The telling of a story can be a container for such an experience. Symbols can represent the healing and growth process as it evolves past symptoms into health and rebirth. Numerous authors have used the term *Hero's Journey* to describe a process in which a person accepts an invitation to this journey and undergoes a series of challenges leading to personal transformation. The process often involves changing habits and thought patterns that impede authenticity while discovering inner truths about oneself and the universe. The metaphor of the hero's journey can give strength, courage, and meaning when an individual is challenged by a serious disease, injury, or a life crisis.

The hero's triumph over these challenges leads to a personal gain, and often a gift to others or to humanity as a whole. *The Lord of the Rings* describes Frodo Baggins' quest to destroy the one ring at Mount Doom. Through his journey he keeps his commitment – sometimes blindly and without knowing how to accomplish it – often at great peril to himself. Yet in the end he saves Middle Earth from the dark forces. And remember: he had help.

Most personal stories are less dramatic on the surface but represent commitment to overcoming adversity with varying degrees of success. It is difficult for most people to see that in the midst of great difficulty, they might be on their own hero's journey.

Some individuals neglect self care until they are desperate and overwhelmed with stress. Others find that practicing one or more of these skills regularly actually decreases stress and improves resilience. Some even say that they just don't get stressed the way they used to get stressed before using some of these techniques.

For those who have learned some self care skills in the past, returning to those may be easier than learning new skills. It may boost incentive to remember the success that came with previously learned activities.

CHAPTER 9

MEDITATION: BENEFITS OF STILLNESS

Being in Stillness

The ability to do energy healing or heal oneself is greatly improved with a regular meditation practice that clears the mind and allows the energy to flow. A simple definition of meditation is *to quiet the mind*. Meditation begins with relaxation, good posture and concentration on the present moment. Even this simple practice, if done regularly, can change brainwaves, create more harmony between brain and heart and mind and body. Meditation decreases stress by promoting the relaxation response: lowering blood pressure, decreasing heart rate, and decreasing metabolic rate. The organs can work more efficiently when blood is not being forced through them at high pressure caused by the stress response. During relaxation tissues can heal, detoxification can occur, immunity is increased, and the body can function more effectively. Note that when individuals are depressed or have certain thought disorders, it is difficult to concentrate and meditation may not be possible.

A female patient in the hospital had fallen on a rocky trail while on vacation. She had an injured shoulder and a collapsed lung and had a chest tube in place. She was sitting in a chair when I arrived. I explained Healing Touch and asked if she did any meditation. She said she did, but her response led me to believe that she had not thought of using meditation to help her current painful situation. I encouraged her to re-connect with her meditation practice during the Healing Touch treatment. During the session I sensed her going deeply into her healing process. I gave her a few more treatments during which she went into her meditation state. She was able to have the chest tube removed a day earlier than expected.

In Quaker teachings and in the Bible, reference is made to connecting with *the still, small voice within.* Meditation can be used to contact *the inner teacher or wise mind.* Being in the stillness is an opportunity to listen. A question sometimes arises about the difference between meditation and prayer. Some say lightheartedly: Prayer is talking to a higher being; meditation is listening.

Regular practice in stillness disciplines the mind to focus and release distractions, allowing inner guidance to surface to conscious awareness. For some, the process of meditation allows the expansion of consciousness until it merges with the infinite. Deep in the subconscious rests all experiences one has had. Meditation can help one get in touch with inner strength as well as release the fears and expectations of the ego. Meditation is a means of sorting out superficial experience from deeper truth. It can be a path to the important words of advice from Socrates: *Know thyself.* Using meditation to gain clarity about one's motivations and agendas will help the healer avoid projecting personal issues onto a client and will also prevent getting tangled up in the client's issues. Listening to inner wisdom, helps one make better decisions or have a better understanding of experiences.

Through meditation a willing mind may be able to access spiritual helpers and guides. These experiences may be a function of the wise mind, personal projections, or beings of a higher vibration. They may appear as angels, saints, beings of light, or aspects of the divine. These helpers may provide guidance or actual assistance in healing if requested to do so. On her audiotape "The Power of Prayer," Joan Borysenko tells a story about a collective of souls who are stuck in a room because they did not know they *could* ask for help.

In a type of meditation called Sat Nam Rasayan, meditators set an intention for themselves or others and then create a *healing space* by raising the vibration with a brief chant and then focusing on their own internal sensations. Energy is not "sent" but instead, the space is held for the healing to occur.

Guided imagery is another way of accessing a meditative state, particularly when the mind is very busy. Imagery or visualization can set up neural pathways in the brain that help accomplish what we imagine such as a relaxed state of being. There are many such recorded guided imagery programs available, and simply listening to the voice of someone leading an imagery session for relaxation and healing can help focus one's thoughts and move the listener through the restless state that sometimes occurs in the early phase of meditation.

Janet Mentgen taught a type of meditation called Yoga Nidra, which is the process of quieting the body while keeping the mind active. Using a Mind Mirror for biofeedback she connected electrodes to a person's scalp, which registered readings of the person's ability to access beta, alpha, theta, and delta waves. Patterns in rows of tiny red lights on a screen showed when a person in meditation was progressing through the different states and whether the left and right hemispheres were synchronized. Observations showed that Yoga Nidra could indeed help the brain access the waves symmetrically, in both the right and left hemispheres.

The process of meditation can also have wider social effects as demonstrated by a study done in 1993. In the study 4000 trained meditators temporarily relocated to Washington DC. They practiced Transcendental Meditation for eight weeks. The crime rate was decreased by 24 percent during the length of the study.

Intention

Intention is the calm focus of one's full attention on the purpose at hand. Intention is not just wishing It is the focus of body, mind, and spirit to carry out a task. Energy follows thought and will go in the direction of one's focused attention to ultimately manifest the intended reality.

Jury duty came for me one stormy winter. A holiday and a snow day off from business caused the session to last extra days. The case was a motor vehicle collision during which a young man was injured. I cringed each time the lawyer for the plaintiff described how gruesomely the man had been injured and how terribly it would affect his life. I could sense the energy of those words working their damage into his energy field. I realized that I may have been selected for the jury so that I could hold a healing intention for him during the trial.

During the third week of the trial the jury started the third day of deliberations. Many hours were being spent going over the same material again and again. Two jurors with opposing opinions insisted they would not change their mind about who caused the accident. We had nearly a dozen issues to decide and were still stuck on the first question.

At one point I had the idea to hold energy for a "shift." I focused on my breath, holding the thought of "shift" while keeping track of the deliberations. I was hoping that some change could re-direct the energy of the discussion. After 45 minutes another female juror suggested that we check with the judge about whether we had to answer the questions in the order listed on the sheet. The judge said we could answer them in any order we wished. We started at the end. The last question on the sheet actually asked about what percent was each of the drivers to blame for the accident. Somehow when each of the disagreeing jurors was able to quantify his opinion as a percentage (and a small one at that), it clarified days of discussion. Each had spoken his piece. The rest of the questions were decided within an hour.

Opinions vary about how to hold an intention during energy work. Some feel it is important to hold the intention tenaciously during the entire treatment while others feel that once stated we can release it and trust the universe as we open to give or receive the healing. As we evolve our consciousness, we can develop the ability to hold a high vibration and a positive intention all the time. This is one way of spreading healing in the world.

Some people have had success using a visual display board with pictures representing their intentions. This type of *vision board* or *treasure map* holds the energy of hopes and dreams and helps maintain a focus – even unconsciously – on achieving the end result.

In *The Secret* (2006: Atria Books), Rhonda Byrnes reveals many examples in which energy follows thought. The secret is the Law of Attraction, through which thoughts attract things, including success in relationships, finances, and health. Positive thoughts have a high vibration that attracts positive outcomes which also have a high vibration. Negative thoughts have a low vibration which attracts vibrations causing negative outcomes.

Joe Vitale wrote several related books, including *The Attraction Factor* (2008, John Wilkey & Sons), in which he states that the Law of Attraction is "always working." He teaches that we merely need to "place our order" with the universe in order to attract our intended outcomes, though he admits that to get it to work we have to clear any unconscious, limiting thoughts or attitudes that block receptivity.

The late Wayne Dyer, who wrote *The Power of Intention* (2005, Hay House), describes intention as an energy of which we are a part. He says it is "the force in the universe that allows the power of creation to take place." When we align with this Source, all things are possible. Working with spirit in this way is referred to as *co-creation*.

Esther and Jerry Hicks' book *Ask and It Is Given* (2008, Hay House) describes the Law of Attraction like this: when we are aligned with Source energy, manifestation of what we want is easy, especially when we add *appreciation* to the process. Hicks explains that appreciation for life and all that surrounds it is the final key in the Law of Attraction. Appreciation encourages everyone to see the world through the eyes of the Source. Esther Hicks is known for her channeling sessions in which a group of entities called *Abraham* speak through her. Many of these sessions are available on YouTube.

Most of the authors above found themselves in financially or emotionally difficult times. They used Intention, or the Laws of Attraction, to move themselves into successful and fulfilling lives.

Lynne McTaggart is another author and researcher who expands the possibilities of intention to worldwide dynamics. She studied the effect that occurs when a large number of people all focus their intention on the same outcome or goal. McTaggert's *The Intention Experiment* (2007, Free Press) documents the effects of group focus. One such experiment involved groups of people successfully meditating to increase plant growth. Another unpublished experiment studied the effects of a group of over ten thousand people holding the intention for peace in Sri Lanka. The reported results showed that although injuries and deaths increased during the brief time of the experiment, they dramatically decreased in the weeks following.

In addition to the observed results, McTaggart also surveyed participants who were holding the peaceful intention during the Sri Lanka experiment. She found that 44% reported improvements in many types of relationships and 38% noticed a difference even in their relationships with strangers. It was as if meditating with thousands of strangers created a bond that enhanced the group's ability to be accepting of people they did not know. This is yet another example of how healing work has dynamic and unexpected benefits to those who provide service to others with little expectation of receiving anything in return.

Intuition

Energy work and meditation tend to open the channel of intuition — the inner wisdom of things known without having been learned. In a world where issues are often so complex that it is impossible to have all the information necessary to gain an accurate understanding of them, intuitive wisdom is valuable for making good decisions. In cases where there is no time and choices must be made instantaneously, intuition is an immediately accessible resource. For example, on 9/11 when planes crashed into the World Trade towers, there were many stories told of people who were spared injury or death due to being late or not getting to work for different reasons. Were they directed by intuition?

Intuition is accessing subtle inner guidance, which is below the surface of one's awareness and is often symbolic and sometimes illogical. Intuition may come in small bits of information over time. Pursuing these trends or patterns can lead to the resolution of a personal issue or receiving guidance toward a new path in life. Intuition can also keep us on task with our true purpose for being on earth. However, intuition is difficult to interpret if it becomes entwined with emotion. Many people receive intuitive information which they ignore or attribute to a lucky guess. Developing intuition may require surrendering one's own desires to a greater wisdom and truly listening.

Developing intuitive skills requires paying attention to experiences with a new focus. A physical sensation or feeling could lead to an awareness that is intuitive. Pay attention to occurrences that seems coincidental or situations that attract your attention for no logical reason at all. Even if ignored, these experiences may provide insights retrospectively. Many people comment after a missed opportunity, "I should have followed my intuition," or "I knew that was going to happen and I could have done something." Occasionally, something in the environment sets off an immediate insight.

Notice how at times you unexpectedly meet people whom you discover can help with a question, project or challenge in your life. Or a friend with whom you want to talk suddenly calls. If you end up somewhere and don't understand why you are there, consider that you may have been brought there to hold energy or to be supportive to someone — whether or not you realize it. Although your behavior is ultimately under your conscious control, following intuition may lead to unexpected insights and meaningful experiences.

Although intuition is at work all of the time, the process of becoming aware of it and using it is enhanced by meditation and silence. Although technological advancements and political events occupy much of current human awareness, the development of intuition seems to hold a great potential for creating honest interactions and an evolved consciousness for all.

Using inner wisdom leads to a deeper spirituality and a deeper connection to all others in the world. Once we completely realize that connection it will be difficult to live without thinking about the impact of our actions on others, no matter how distant or isolated from us they may be.

Following one's intuition can lead to unexpected events that are sometimes explained as synchronicity or serendipity, such as in the following example:

Some years ago I went to have some repairs on my vehicle. The mechanic's office was in a small trailer. After a few comments about the repairs, the man asked what work I did. I hesitated, letting my intuition help me decide whether or not to describe the healing work I do. When I told him about energy work he nodded, paused, and then said he had something to show me on the computer.

It was a story of premature twin girls that had circulated on the internet. One of the babies was doing poorly. Against rules and accepted practice, but most likely following intuition, a nurse put the healthy twin in the bassinette facing her ill sister. The picture showed the healthy twin's arm reaching over and holding the more vulnerable twin. As the story went, the weaker sister began to stabilize as vital signs improved while being held in the energy of her sister.

I had a sense that taking a risk to share about my work opened the door to this man sharing the inspiring article. It reinforced my sense of the importance of trusting inner wisdom, as I did with this car repair person and as the nurse in the story did with caring for her tiny patients.

Meditation is a discipline that enhances the ability to hold an intention. It also helps access inner wisdom or intuition. Being able to hold intentions and access intuition can help whether confronted with difficult life situations, working with clients who have challenging needs for healing, connecting with others, or staying on track with one's life purpose.

CHAPTER 10

LIFE TRANSITIONS
AND DEATH

The sacred transition at the end of life is a time when energy healing can provide support to the dying individual as well as to others present. Family and friends are often at a loss for what to do or say, or may have unresolved issues that create struggle. Healing Touch in general offers a profound peacefulness and even a particular technique for transitions, so all concerned are better able to be present and relaxed. Here are some examples of how Healing Touch has been utilized during these transitional times.

A friend, Debbie, was a hospice volunteer, visiting an individual who was dying. Several family members were present, arguing and shouting at each other. Debbie offered Healing Touch to each family member. They became civil and caring toward one another.

After finishing a Healing Touch session with one patient at the hospital, I asked the nurses if there were any other patients who might be interested in a treatment. One nurse said there was a man dying of cancer and I could ask his family about giving him a treatment. Soon the daughter walked in and was glad to help me give her father Healing Touch. He was unresponsive, but we explained out loud to him what we were offering and let him know it might help decrease any pain he was having. We took a moment to intuitively listen for whether it was alright with him. She and I both had a sense that he gave permission. As we did the technique for transitions, I guided the daughter to each hand position and movement. The patient continued to be unresponsive.

Next I offered the same technique to the daughter, since family members also experience a major transition when a loved one is dying. The daughter, who had been awake all night, sat in a chair resting while receiving the energy healing.

By then the patient's wife had walked in and I offered her a session for her support. The daughter had left and returned, telling me the hospice workers would be doing an assessment for hospice care and helping move the patient back home. She asked them to wait until the mother's session was finished.

After the sessions I left the room grateful that I was able to offer support to this family at a special time. A few minutes later a hospital staff member informed me that the patient had died. It seemed that the death occurred at a time of peacefulness for the patient and family, and the patient was spared the discomfort of being moved back to his home.

I later reflected on the timing of this experience. I had not been called to see this patient initially. I arrived at the hospital at a time that suited my own schedule and otherwise seemed random. Yet, to be there when the daughter and wife arrived and to have been able to complete those three sessions in the brief time before the man's death seemed more than coincidental and was perhaps guided by some greater force.

The nurses at the hospital requested that I offer Healing Touch to a man who had a leg ulcer, a possible complication from diabetes. The man was middle aged and did not appear very ill. I knew little about him, but was told his wife was a nurse and he did not like doctors. He was however agreeable to some alternative healing.

My assessment revealed that his energy field was depleted. I began the treatment using light touch on his ankle and knee to begin balancing his field. He immediately said, "You have to stop. It's too much." I replied that I could do something else and switched to Hands in Motion without touching. He was agreeable to have me continue without touching, and even commented about how relaxed he felt. Then I had an intuitive idea to do a Healing Touch technique used specifically for transitions.

I completed the technique and he continued to relax and then dozed off. When I returned the next day to offer another treatment, he was being wheeled out of his room on a stretcher to go to the cardiac care unit. His color was ashen and he looked close to death. Because he needed medical attention, I was not able to give him a treatment that day. He died that night. Later, I sensed that his agenda was to get healthcare "over his dead body." I also sensed that perhaps I was brought there to help him make the transition to the next life.

From Lynn Thompson

My nine year old step-daughter, Lyra, had cancer. We were told that once her breathing became labored her transition could take as long as four days. One morning she was having trouble breathing. I thought about calling a friend and Healing Touch practitioner to come and work on her but I thought, "No, I'm trained in acupressure. I will work on her myself." In the past I had been reluctant to do that, maybe because it is so intense to work on family; maybe because I thought her soul wanted to go Home. I did Soul Lightening Acupressure on her. She made her transition about an hour after that. Later a psychic friend of mine who was in touch with her from the Other Side said she thanked me for it.

In my own family, I had this experience:

On a visit to my mother in Buffalo a few years ago, it was obvious that she was beginning a major transition at age 86. She was confused at times and not functioning well, after being healthy, lucid, and independent and her whole life. Mom had clear moments during which she talked about being ready to die. After the days of visiting and planning her care with siblings, I went home to Alaska to take care of some issues and planned to return to stay with her indefinitely. While back in Alaska, I met with a monthly intention meditation group scheduled at my office. During my turn for the group to hold my intention, I set the intention for my mother to resolve whatever was needed so she could die with grace and ease. I felt very connected to her during the meditation. After the group I listened to a phone message from my sister saying that mom had died. Later I realized that she passed away during the exact time when we were holding energy for her. Oddly, it was the only time that a caretaker had not been with her in the three weeks during or after my visit.

Yet, I felt that I was with her in an energetic and spiritual way. I felt honored to be part of her transition.

Death tends to bring a great deal of emotion to the surface. Even individuals who have accepted that a terminally ill loved one will pass, must deal with the finality of death when it actually occurs. Others may have mixed feelings arise from unresolved anger, vulnerabilities from relationships, and dreams that will never be realized. Healing Touch and other energy modalities provide a sense of peace through a sometimes daunting, though sacred time.

CHAPTER 11

TRAUMA:
EXPERIENCE AND HEALING

Trauma Experience

The prevalence of trauma of all types is widespread throughout much of the world and includes trauma from accident, child abuse and neglect, domestic violence, political conflict, war, or other human struggles. The many faces of bullying, hatred, economic insecurity and oppression (racism, sexism) leave a steady stream of survivors carrying the burdens of fear, anxiety, rage, and physical illness.

The effects of trauma on the functioning of the brain is an expanding subject of research and treatment. Trauma can change the chemistry of the brain and disrupt normal human functioning. Information in this section has been taken from the works of Judith Lewis Hermann, MD, Robert Scaer, MD, Peter Levine, PhD, and Belleruth Naparstek, LISW, BCD.

These authors have defined trauma as the real or perceived threat to one's life or sense of well-being. The results of trauma can be physical, emotional, cognitive, social, economic, and spiritual. The impact of trauma is layered in the neurological and endocrine system, affecting all parts of the body and mind. Life force energy can become blocked. There might be physical injury as well as chronic pain syndromes or immune problems that occur from long term stress. Emotions or unmet needs can become stuck, leaving the person trapped in patterns of thought, emotion, or behavior. Trauma also makes individuals more vulnerable to further stressors.

Intergenerational trauma occurs when the unresolved and unhealed trauma of one generation is passed to the next generation. For example, traumatized individuals who become parents may have poor coping skills and other symptoms of Post Traumatic Stress Disorder (PTSD) which can have adverse effects on their children. Shared experience of being victimized by racism and/or other oppressions and socio-cultural disadvantages increases the likelihood of intergenerational trauma effects.

Discovering how these changes are actually occurring physically, the study of epigenetics is revealing that certain methyl molecules that attach to DNA during trauma can biochemically transmit the effects of trauma to the next generation (Szyf and Meany). While the DNA itself is not changed, these molecules change the environment of the DNA which can alter its expression. It is known, too, that the environment of the DNA can also be changed by diet, lifestyle, and perhaps attitude.

In times of danger, parts of the hormonal system are activated in order to help mobilize a person for survival and safety. Stress hormones increase heart rate and breathing and shunt blood to muscles and away from digestive organs. The conscious thought process is shut down so that unconscious survival reflexes take control over behavior. The stress hormones such as epinephrine (adrenalin) are usually discharged as a person takes action with the *fight or flight* response and the body returns to normal functioning.

However, in some situations the person is not able to fight or get away. He or she might be held captive or otherwise helpless, and instead experience the *freeze* response in which the stress hormones continue to circulate, stimulating the neurons to keep firing as if responding to stress. In situations of extreme trauma or unpredictable trauma over time, the nervous system remains in a trauma state disrupting the normal balance of the body. As a result, resilience is decreased. This chemical pattern causes the survivor of the trauma to feel and act as if the traumatic event is never over.

Following severe trauma, the stress response may become triggered or activated with cues from the environment that are only mildly related to the trauma. This *kindling* response leaves the survivor vulnerable to being triggered by a wide range of situations or internal cues that result in chronic anxiety or panic attacks. Chronic illness can result from the body being in the state of frequent or constant alarm. Conditions such as chronic fatigue syndrome, fibromyalgia, chronic pain, endocrine and immune disorders, and other similar illnesses are not unusual for trauma survivors.

Trauma leaves an energetic imprint on the field and inhibits the natural flow of energy, causing a range of problems. However, energy healing can be helpful in clearing the residue of the experience from the energy field and re-balancing the field. Depending on the severity of the trauma, many treatments may be needed.

Healing Trauma

Psychotherapy and counseling may help recovery, especially if a person is able to talk about their feelings and experiences without being re-traumatized. Medications may be needed to stabilize symptoms of depression, anxiety, pain, and chronic illness, so that other recovery work can take place. Medications may be important if a person is unable to function due to the severity of his or her response to trauma.

Support groups offer opportunities where individuals can share their pain with others who have had similar experiences, as well as re-connect with others as recovery progresses. The devastation of trauma often includes falling into substance abuse to escape the torment of ongoing feelings and memories. When addictions become a way of coping, Twelve Step programs have shown that a support group and consistently taking action to help oneself can be life changing.

There are many alternative approaches to healing trauma. Weaving traditional Native American cultural healing practices such as talking circles and drumming into recovery programs can help individuals and groups re-connect to community and develop a new sense of meaning and purpose in their lives. Trauma may leave the individual feeling isolated and alone; re-integration with community is part of the healing.

Holistic approaches using energy healing and self care are useful for the long term process of healing from trauma. Preliminary research with active military returning from Afghanistan showed that a combination of guided imagery and Healing Touch was effective at reducing PTSD and related symptoms, including cynicism, depression, and hostility (Jain, et al). In this study the Guided Imagery tape called *Healing Trauma* (1999) by Naparstek was used.

Counseling and energy healing used concurrently can work as a powerful dual approach. Keeping one's energy field in balance helps stabilize emotional and physical health between counseling sessions. Healing Touch also offers specific techniques for trauma release, pain relief, deep clearing of the energetic residues of trauma, rebalancing the field, and making transitions such as returning to a normalized healthy life. As issues are brought up in therapy sessions, the energy work in separate sessions can clear and re-balance the energy field. The release of emotions during an energy healing session may include crying, laughter, anger, and/or physical movements. Healing Touch techniques can help release the effects of trauma even if an individual is unable to talk about his or her feelings.

Some clients who have experienced trauma are particularly sensitive to issues related to touch and loss of control. Healing Touch treatments can be done without physical contact and provides the client with a choice about when and how much touch is therapeutic.

EFT (tapping acupressure meridians) is sometimes called the *tearless trauma technique* and can be used for every aspect of trauma including memories, emotions, anxiety, addictions, insomnia, physical symptoms, spiritual disconnection, and many other symptoms. One can start the work gently and take gradual steps as the person feels safe enough to go deeper. For example, if specific memories are too overwhelming, tapping on a general phrase such as "something happened" can prevent a person from being painfully triggered. Working with an experienced EFT practitioner who can provide safety and support in the process is helpful.

Here are some examples of how energy approaches show promise in helping survivors release the energy of the trauma and make progress in recovery:

Leah, a Healing Touch Practitioner, received a trauma release treatment from Janet Mentgen in a Healing Touch Advance practice class weeks after a motor vehicle accident. Prior to the treatment she could not move her arm above her shoulder. After the treatment she could extend her arm all the way above her head.

A woman was hospitalized after being mauled by a bear. She had severe injuries to her leg, requiring grafts that were harvested from her other leg. Both sites were painful. She experienced flashbacks from the attack and her sleep was poor. Antibiotics given to prevent infections caused her to have intestinal side effects. She was given numerous Healing Touch treatments during her seven weeks in the hospital. She shared that the treatments helped tremendously, beginning with helping her sleep while in critical care. "Each session left me totally relaxed and free of tension. This was an extreme treat since I'm one of those people who seldom completely relaxes. The hospital environment is not the ideal place for relaxation. I looked forward to my sessions...following a couple sessions there was noticeable reduction in the level of pain I was enduring. This was also a treat!"

There are many other such examples where energy work has helped survivors of mild to severe trauma. Decades ago a few preliminary case studies showed that sexual assault survivors who received Healing Touch after the trauma experience were less likely to have severe PTSD.

On one of his training CD's, Gary Craig, EFT founder and teacher, demonstrated the effects of EFT on severely disabled Viet Nam veterans who had required long term institutionalization. Following a week of EFT treatment, some were able to release the internalized horrors from the war, and re-stabilize.

Interoception: Going Within for Self-Healing

Interoception is the process of consciously paying attention to internal sensations, an ability which may be damaged during the experience of trauma. In a healthy balanced individual these sensations alert one to basic needs such as hunger, when to stop eating, thirst, the need for rest, taking breaks and sleep, as well as when to urinate and defecate. These subtle sensations are imminently valuable for self-regulation and survival. They also give us an awareness of danger. Yet many individuals are disconnected from internal cues due to trauma, stress, or busy lifestyles. There are many unfortunate results including overeating, chronic dehydration, insomnia, addictions, digestion and elimination problems, inflammation, and infections. Many of these conditions are preventable by simply paying attention and responding to the messages from the body.

The simple technique of paying attention to physical sensations has been embedded in many ancient teachings, such as Buddhist mindfulness, and is re-appearing in many practices such as Sat Nam Rasayan (Yogi Bhajan), The Wonder Method (Alain Heriott), and Focusing (Eugene Gendlin). It is interesting to think of how often healers have used the suggestion of "going within" to lead meditations. The practice of interoception is one way to discover and enter this inner space.

Peter Levine's book, *In An Unspoken Voice,* states that the physiological reason that interoception is effective may be due to the function of the vagus nerve, a cranial nerve with an 80% sensory capacity that sends information from the internal organs to the brain. During a state of stress, the brain receives messages about changes that are occurring in the body and interprets them through the limbic, or emotional part of the brain. Increased heart rate and breathing due to stress triggers the emotions to stimulate the stress reaction in the body. For someone who has been traumatized, feeling these stressful sensations in the body can unconsciously cause a trauma response, resulting in severe anxiety and panic. However, when one can pay attention to sensations with a neutral mind and learn that the sensations are transient, it is possible to decrease the hyper-arousal that troubles many survivors. It is important to note that severely traumatized individuals may be triggered by focusing on their physical sensations and should use this approach with a well-trained therapist who can help clients explore fear and be creative in moving through it.

Joan Halifax, a Buddhist teacher and Zen priest, discussed interoception at the Healing Beyond Borders annual conference in Colorado Springs in August 2014. She had worked with neuroscientists who were able to show that when a person pays attention to their internal sensations, the neurons fire in the same part of the brain as when they are being empathetic. Interoceptivity and empathy seem to overlap. In other words, the same mechanism for sensing ourselves may help us to be sensitive to others.

Although the workings of the human body are far more complicated than presented here, the practice of interoception, that is, sitting in stillness and noticing internal sensations with a neutral perspective, is a simple and valuable form of managing stress, creating a coherent state, and helping to heal ourselves and others.

The self care options in this book offer a wide variety of choices for helping oneself. However, when trauma occurs at the hands of another person or when it is so serious that it disrupts day-to-day functioning, it is important to re-establish social connections by building deep and trusting relationships with support groups, therapists, or friends in order to fully recover one's wholeness.

CHAPTER 12

DISTANCE HEALING APPROACHES

Non-Local Energy Work

The practice of energy healing can have an effect even when the client is not present. This approach has been referred to as distance healing, remote healing, absent healing, or non-local healing. It involves intention and, in some cases, using hands-on techniques on oneself or another as a surrogate. Meditation, intention, and prayer are all used to benefit someone's well-being at a distance. Daniel J. Benor MD, in his Article *Distant Healing*, reviewed 61 studies of distance healing on humans, plants, yeast, bacteria, and cells, as well as over 100 cases of healing using hands near the body.

Techniques for Distance Healing

There are different opinions about whether it is necessary to ask permission when giving a distance energy treatment to someone. Having respect for the recipient means giving them a choice. It is also likely that when a person knows about the treatment he or she can be more receptive and possibly have a better outcome. If it is not possible to get permission, one can ask in a spiritual way if the potential client is agreeable, and carefully listen intuitively for the answer. I have heard about a few cases where the clients were focused in another process and it was not a good time for them to receive energy work. This is something to consider when planning a distance healing session. It is also important to set the intention for the highest good to keep one's own agenda from interfering. One might add an intention for the client to receive whatever is needed from the treatment, which also acknowledges that they might not want/ need the session at the time. Keep in mind that our thoughts are always transmitting. We generally don't get someone's permission to verbalize an affirmation for their health, say a prayer, or wish them well in our mind.

Some techniques for Distance Healing;

- Intention. Focusing of the mind by holding positive thoughts for the well-being or highest good of the recipient.
- Presence. By bringing one's awareness into the moment, it is possible to create a vibration for the healing to occur.
- Surrogate. A treatment is given in which the client and practitioner both intend the healing to be directed to a third party who is not present.
- Holding one's hands together close if holding the issue or person between the palms and directing energy or intention for their benefit.
- Photograph. Holding a photo of the recipient between one's hands or in one's presence with the intention of directing the healing energy to the distant recipient.
- Imagery. One can imagine surrounding the client in white light or a healing vibration. Sense the client experiencing harmony and peace. Hold an intention for his or her highest good. Remember, we do not always know exactly what a client needs. Cells and organisms have their own healing wisdom and ability and it is best to support them in a holistic way.
- Ho'Oponopono. This Hawaiian approach involves setting an intention and then saying four sentences: *I love you. I'm sorry. Please forgive me. Thank you.* Once the intention is set, these statements are made to no one in particular but out to the universe in general. They have the effect of erasing from human consciousness the

symptom or troublesome issue (*Zero Limits*, Dr. Ihaleakala Hew Len and Joe Vitale, 2007). As with all culturally based techniques, be aware that this technique is only a tiny slice of healing practices from the Hawaiian culture.

- Prayer. Invoking the supernatural power from one's personal belief system or religious training.

- Affirmations. Positive statements directed toward a person's healing. For example: "My client has the ability to heal completely for the highest good."

- Intentions can be used for healing the environment or for the resolution of destructive conflicts in the world. This can bring us into vibration with many others who are holding this same intention. It may be that some conflicts will only shift when they are brought into a higher vibration.

- Reiki (Mikao Usui) and Mari-El (Ethel Lombardi) are both energy healing modalities which have specific symbols for distance healing. The symbols can be traced on the healer's hands or held in the healer's thoughts while directing a healing intention toward the client. The symbols provide a vibration for the healing to be done.

Here are some examples of healing-at-a-distance in action:

A friend Sue, who lived several blocks away, described having fatigue, headache and oncoming cold symptoms while we were on the phone. I told her I would give her a distance Healing Touch treatment after we got off the phone. Although I had good intentions, I was finishing a task and did not start the treatment for 40 minutes or so. The treatment took about 30 minutes. Almost immediately after I finished, Sue called to tell me her headache was gone and she felt well-enough to do things she needed to do. She did not know when I started or finished, but she reported feeling better after I had finished.

A number of years ago I received a summons for a legal deposition. I was a bit nervous about it since I had not had experience giving testimony as a witness before. I emailed Healing Touch friends and acquaintances and asked for their energetic support by keeping me in their intentions and meditations. I believe

I received help from them because I was amazingly calm and relaxed and felt confident while answering hours of questions from several lawyers in the room.

I offered my sister a distance Healing Touch treatment on her birthday one year. She said her chronic shoulder problem had been causing pain. I encouraged her to rest while she received the treatment from me thousands of miles away. She later told me that it helped a lot and she was in less pain after the treatment.

CHAPTER 13

TRANSFORMATION

Personal Evolution

No matter what motivation brings a person to an energy work class, a treatment, or meditation, experiencing universal healing energy can open a person to sometimes unexpected changes. Since the work transcends linear reality, personal transformations can happen over time or suddenly.

Time and again, as a Healing Touch instructor, I see that even in a beginning energy class individuals experience a shift in their personal awareness and are forever changed with a new ability of perceiving. In that way, the basics of energy healing can be a springboard to a new consciousness and the tipping point to the next stage in evolution.

Many problems for which people seek counseling are spiritual problems needing spiritual direction. In his book *Joy's Way (1979)*, Dr. Brugh Joy describes Transformational Psychology as a path for helping the client change focus from a mental perception of a problem to awareness from a deeper consciousness. The role of a transformational therapist is to determine where the soul is going and to help remove the blocks to its getting there; or in other words, to encourage the client to be true to their soul. When these blocks are surpassed, wonderful new experiences can come into awareness and life can take on a quality that may have been previously obscured or minimized.

For many the changes are subtle. Individuals may notice that when opportunities arise for more spiritually related activities, they have a tendency to choose those activities, whether a class, a movie, receiving a treatment, or participating in a conversation. For others who tend to attract or create more drama, the transitions may feel like a whirlwind of relationship beginnings or endings, family upheavals, altered employment conditions, personal realizations, or health issues. Some people interpret these seemingly out-of-control and often painful situations as the exact turn of events needed to open their thinking or provide new choices in behavior, leading to a whole new experience of life. A community of people who are going through similar experiences can offer support and share wisdom. Having a place to talk about the impact of these events can help to find meaning in these experiences and to feel that we are not alone with them.

One friend and colleague, Diane Wind Wardell, PhD, RN, described her changes this way:

It is a long journey and one that keeps evolving as I walk quietly down its path. Not that it was always quiet! In the early days of learning Healing Touch my personal changes created quite a bit of disturbance in my family. So much so that my youngest son, when asked what he wanted for Christmas, asked for his "old mother back". Stepping into my new awareness of recognizing myself as somehow different I asked what she, this "old mother" was like. He responded with, "she was more judgmental, got angrier easier, well....you know....never mind, you can stay." And I did. I stayed in a place of reflection and growth. That "old mother" is still there on some days and it gives me a chance to work through my issues again. In truth, it is really again and again and again! But, I am ever different.

Healing Touch classes generate a lot of energy. In that setting the group is generally able to hold the amount of energy needed to create deeper experiences. *In one class, a student had had a metal plate in her head for thirty years. The area on her head was so sensitive that she could not even let the hairdresser touch her head. After a session given to her during a level 2 class, she no longer has problems with her head being touched.*

For myself personally, I know that my life changed within the first hour of a Healing Touch class. Other related classes and meditations had cracked a door open, but now the door was flung wide open. Even with limited experience I could feel a sense of integration and expansion among many aspects of myself including my awareness of spirituality and intuition, my love of nature and being outdoors, my social self, and my professional work as a psychiatric nurse. Having those compartments brought together felt wonderful.

Long ago, a woman in a Healing Touch class shared that she previously belonged to a fundamentalist religion. I was curious about this seemingly unlikely shift to embracing energy healing. When I asked her about it, she replied, "My idea of God just kept getting bigger."

Another woman was in the hospital for respiratory problems. I explained the treatment and helped her get comfortable. I asked if she had any spiritual beliefs that could help her in her healing process. She said there wasn't anything in particular and closed her eyes to begin relaxing. As the session started she began to tell me a story about a relative whose child had seizures. The child's mother was taking the boy to a medical facility in another location for evaluation. As the story was told, once they were in the big city, the mother cautioned the child to be careful because they were no longer in their small town. Although the mother had been advised by friends in the hometown to use reputable cab companies for her travel in the city, a desk clerk where they were staying called a taxi from an unfamiliar company. As things happened, the son ended up in the front seat with the cab driver. The mother could not hear all the conversation, but the driver seemed kind and the child was interested in the conversation with him. As they got out of the cab, she found the cab driver extremely courteous and helpful with their bags. She took note of the number of the taxi.

When the tests were completed, the mother received a report that there were no signs of lesions in her son's brain. She thought back on the cab driver and wanted to thank him. When she called the taxi company to try to thank the man, she was told there was no taxi with that number in their small fleet and no driver that fit the description she gave. She wondered how it all fit together…her son's conversation with the cab driver, negative test results, and mysteriously not finding that cab driver.

From Lynn Thompson:

Here is another story — this one is about how I got started doing Soul Lightening Acupressure. I was at a class in Cranio-Sacral therapy. In the same hotel a class in SEVA Stress Release (a Soul Lightening protocol) was being taught. The students did a demonstration on us. I was amazed at how the work made my body feel - and they had had only two days training. The most remarkable thing was that the White Light got in my face and said, "This is what you're going to do."

When giving an energy healing treatment to another person, the focus is on their needs and what can be done to help. Yet the very process of moving into alignment with spirit, becoming still and centered, and acting in the interest of another is likely to help the healer as well. Participating in this connection with another validates our humanity and allows us to feel full and whole in a way that may be rare. For many, even good relationships have many demands and expectations to manage, whereas energy healing can transcend worldly agendas.

Energy healing can become a lifestyle when one strives to live a spiritual life and maintain continuous alignment with Source energy. For those interested in becoming healers, Janet Mentgen recommended doing something each day that is related to healing: meditate, read, give energy treatments, hold a healing intention, live with purpose, and stay connected with spirit.

A sense of community and interaction with other energy workers seems to help keep us on track when the demands of living in the world distract us from this purpose. Janet's far-reaching vision built an international community of healers not only connected to each other for mutual support and growth, but also connected to the world.

Perhaps the abilities discussed in this book are like other developments in the human race: at first there are a few who possess a new awareness, and then the capacity spreads, like the allegory of the hundredth monkey. At this time in history we regard a few people as being psychic, intuitive, or having healing abilities. People who can attract resources easily might be considered *lucky.* But what if we are all meant to have access to more abilities? I believe that these expanded faculties are qualities of our true selves, waiting just beneath the surface. We may only need to release our resistance.

Social Change

It will be a powerful sign of social transformation when we routinely hear about energy healing and heart-centered conflict resolution in the public media. How inspiring it could be to hear statistics about illness and stress declining as more people move into states of balanced energy. Although programs exist for children to have relaxation or structured self-control time, it would be a benefit for society to have these programs be widespread in schools, and workplaces. Incorporating energy healing into patient care in health care facilities would add an extra dimension to the comfort, healing process, and prevention of illness for many people.

CHAPTER 14

HISTORY, SCIENCE, AND SOCIAL PERSPECTIVES IN ENERGY HEALING

A New Consciousness

Many events in the past century have provided a background for the development of holistic awareness in Western culture. Holistic principles which address body, mind, and spirit created a framework for the emergence of energy healing.

For example, over 100 years ago, American theosophists studied the mysteries of the divine and its relationship to nature and humans, embracing Eastern philosophies to gain a deeper spirituality. During this time Hinduism was introduced to the West. Decades later, the expulsion of the Dalai Lama from Tibet resulted in Buddhist wisdom and practice spreading to more parts of the world.

The 20th century continued to unfold with two world wars, harnessing of nuclear power, the Viet Nam war, the legal end of apartheid, the tearing down of the Berlin Wall, terrorism, and tremendous advances in technology, including developments which make it possible to explore space or to have the world linked by communications networks. Amidst these changes music and culture also took new directions. In 1967 the musical *Hair* announced *"The dawning of the Age of Aquarius."* Institutions such as Esalen and spiritual and ecological communities such as Findhorn in Scotland and Damanhur in Italy were founded to promote expanding consciousness, spirituality, and sustainability. In 1980 Marilyn Ferguson wrote a book called *The Aquarian Conspiracy* describing new possibilities for how we can evolve as humans. In 1987 the *Harmonic Convergence* celebrated the first globally synchronized meditation, which took place at the time of an alignment of planets in our solar system.

As these and other events have unfolded, many individuals and groups have gravitated toward optimism and hopefulness. They have a sense of synchronicity and see everything as connected. Many are inspired to find meaning and purpose in their lives and are joining with others to find commonalities. In the face of natural and human-made disasters, many hold on to a sense of community to prevent social disintegration. Defending human rights is now an international endeavor.

Some children are being born with more spiritual awareness. These *Indigo* children, as they are sometimes called, grow to question political and social assumptions. If their skills and perceptions are nurtured, they may be the ones to lead the way out of political strife and poverty. One seventeen-year-old female who was interviewed by Oprah Winfrey in a video called *About Us: The Dignity of Children* (1997) shared an insight from her own consciousness: "I don't think people will evolve individually, I think we are going to do it in groups."

These are but a few examples of events and experiences causing and expressing shifts in human awareness. Science, spirituality, philosophy, and many other areas of thinking continue to open as consciousness expands and we see what we are capable of achieving.

The science fiction book *Strands* (2014) describes an increase in human capacity based on the possibility of evolving DNA – that is, from the double helix of two strands to a new structure of twelve strands. In the novel a character experiences an acute sharpening of the senses and is able to see the rings around Saturn without artificial lenses. The novel also puts forth the idea that humans with more DNA could have an enhanced ability to heal themselves, even to the point of organ and limb regeneration. Some of the characters in the book can communicate spiritually and intuitively with each other through a web of energy surrounding the planet, with no technological assistance. The novel describes how the ability for people to genuinely care about one another promotes decisions that show a respect for the entire population as well as the earth. Though much of science fiction has often come across as "unbelievable" at first, much of it also comes to pass. Many of the changes described in *Strands* are already happening.

Body-Mind Medicine Examples in Literature

Energy healing is considered just one of many holistic approaches. Over the years much has been learned about the interactions of body and mind, resulting in many body/mind approaches to healing. Decades ago Hans Selye PhD reported the effects of stress on the body in his *General Adaptation Theory.* Herb Benson MD later showed the effects of the *relaxation response* for healing. In the book *Mind Body Medicine: How to Use Your Mind for Better Health*, Daniel Goleman MD, highlighted the power of the mind in examples using meditation and imagery in healing. In reviewing numerous studies in relaxation, imagery, hypnosis, positive thinking, biofeedback, exercise, and mindfulness, he found that these approaches were helpful in healing many common conditions including heart disease, skin and digestive disorders, and immune problems. In *Biology of Belief,* Bruce Lipton described how thoughts and emotions alter the receptivity of cell membranes, causing the cells to function differently depending on how a person feels. Elizabeth Blackburn won a Nobel Prize in 2014 for showing that meditation can lengthen telomeres at the end of the DNA strand, which are associated with healthier aging.

In her book *The Heart Speaks,* Mimi Guarneri MD, describes how cynicism and hostility increase symptoms of heart disease, such as increased heart rate, blood pressure, production of epinephrine, and other chemicals that might be responsible for arterial wall thickening. She discusses how angry thoughts increase arousal of the fight or flight response and may become a chronic state for some. Others are diagnosed with stress-induced heart failure, in which intense emotional pain brings symptoms of chest pain, shortness of breath, and heart muscle weakness. Dr. Guarneri refers to this form of stress cardiomyopathy as *broken heart syndrome,* since it sometimes occurs in patients who have a serious loss. It is also well documented that depression increases the risk of death after a heart attack, while group support, as well as love, forgiveness, optimism, and gratitude promote health and recovery.

In *The Inflammation Cure,* William Joel Meggs MD, PhD, describes how thoughts can cause physical responses in our bodies: "Our thoughts, stress levels, moods, and even social lives can trigger a cascade of inflammatory reactions in our bodies that could lead to heart disease, asthma, or other health problems."

More evidence of the body-mind connection is demonstrated by the placebo effect. For example, in some tests subjects receiving a substance with no pain relieving properties reported experiencing diminished pain after being told that the substance was a pain reliever.

This placebo effect was even more dramatic when knee surgery patients in Finland were given operations that involved no actual correction to their knee cartilage problems. All patients agreed to participate in the study knowing they might or might not have the damaged parts of the meniscus removed. The non-correction group having only had superficial incisions reported nearly as much improvement to knee function as the corrective surgery recipients. A year later, even the minor benefit of less pain after exercise was no longer evident for the corrective surgery patients.

The opposite of a placebo effect has been shown in *nocebo* experiments. When recipients were given a substance with no active properties, but told it had side effects, they felt sick. In another study, participants allowed their skin to be touched by a non-poisonous plant they thought was poisonous. Again, the belief caused them to exhibit skin reactions. These are only a few examples of the body-mind connection that can be directed to help each person's healing process.

Historical Perspectives

In earlier cultures, shamans and specially delegated individuals functioned in the role of healers. Shamans and other healers passed on their skills through lengthy apprenticeships. Some modern healing traditions still use the process of apprenticeship for teaching skills. An apprentice may need years of study in order to peel away old patterns of thinking that interfere with learning new skills. When this "peeling away" reaches a certain stage, the apprentice can then develop a different relationship with time and space in which these new special skills can be put to use.

Though energy work is new to the West, many older cultures have had an understanding of the energy field for quite some time. Several Asian traditions use the words Chi, Ki, or Qi to describe this energy. Qi Gong, a balancing of the forces called Yin and Yang, is the basis of thousands of years of Chinese medicine. In the Hindu tradition the life force is referred to as Prana; a related healing approach is called Pranic Healing. Ancient practices of Shamanism still use chanting, drumming, dancing, fasting, imagery, and rituals to shift energy for the purpose of healing. A shaman can connect directly with nature in order to bring harmony to an individual, a tribe, a group of people, or even a physical location in need of clearing, balance or a change of energy.

In early Christian art, paintings showed energy radiating around the head (or around the entire body) of certain Saints and revered individuals. These energy fields were referred to as "halos." In these traditions the word *grace* is used to describe this state of balance or being blessed. Being in the *state of grace* might be interpreted to mean that the person has attained a connection to the supernatural or has achieved high energy frequency or an awesome state of balance and harmony.

Bridging Science and Spirituality

In the 1600's the philosophy of cartesian dualism held that the body and mind were separate. Much in Western medical practice has been influenced by the idea of that separation. The body was seen as a machine and the goal of treatment was simply to fix a broken part. Holistic practice seeks to re-establish the principle of wholeness for health.

The subtle energy involved in healing work is invisible to most people. It is a challenge to describe and understand it. Yet, many who study energy agree that everything is made of energy. In the words of physicist Max Planck, "All matter originates and exists only by virtue of a force. We must assume behind this force the existence of a conscious and intelligent Mind. This Mind is the matrix of all matter."

Various definitions of *energy* describe it as a force, available power, the ability to do work, or capacity to produce movement or change. Energy is the life force that maintains the physical processes to keep the body alive. The Human Energy Field holds thoughts, emotions, and the spiritual vibrations of our being. Greg Braden, a scientist and researcher of healing, uses a spiritual term to describe energy. He calls the energy field the *Divine Matrix*. Scientific research has not yet resolved the question of the origin of the life force. At this time, a number of scientists acknowledge that in this area we are exploring the realm of the mystical.

Energy Healing Research

Many scientific studies have been conducted to test the efficacy of holistic practices. The Heart Math Institute is one bridge between science and healing. Heart Math scientists have studied the effect of certain mental exercises on heart rate variability for the purpose of determining the extent to which the heart and brain influence each other, for better or for worse. The Heart Math practices involve an awareness of stressful emotions, slowing the breath, and using positive imagination and affirmative statements. According to the Heart Math Institute, *coherence* is an optimal state of functioning which results when the heart and brain work in harmony. Coherent energy patterns can reorganize discordant energy and bring about healing as a result.

Healing Touch studies have shown many promising results, including reduction of pain and anxiety (Healing Touch Research Survey, A Publication of Healing Touch International, Inc, 2010). One such study followed women receiving radiation treatment for cancer. As a result of Healing Touch, they reported less fatigue, less depression, less anxiety and a better quality of life. Healing Touch given before biopsy procedures reduced anxiety, an effect that for some lasted into the next day. Respiratory and blood pressure rates were also reduced in the same participants. Leukemia patients in another study reported less fatigue and nausea.

A study of patients after coronary artery bypass surgery showed a decrease in anxiety scores as well as shorter length of stays in outpatient treatment (MacIntyre, et al. 2005). Numerous studies have been conducted with similar results.

Also available is the Healing Touch Research Brief: A Summary of Topics on Research and Strategies for the Future, 2015 Edition, a publication of Healing Beyond Borders (HealingBeyondBorders.org).

The Quantum Realm

Much remains to be studied in order to prove the processes by which energy healing actually works. The past century has seen scientific frameworks expand to include theories in the new science of quantum physics, which seeks to describe the energy and behavior of the tiniest known particles. These theories are beginning to provide possible explanations for the various phenomena experienced in energy healing. Quantum physics has not yet achieved the goal of discovering a unifying theory of everything, but so far, it has provided theories that when proven may eventually explain the dynamics of energy healing.

From quantum physics we learn that the smallest known bit of matter is both a wave and a particle, each manifesting under certain conditions. Quantum physics indicates that matter comes into existence when the energy waves collapse into particles, According to this theory, energy precedes matter. Energy healers understand that thoughts and symptoms exist in the energy field before they manifest in the body. It is possible then, to clear these disturbances from the energy field before they become symptoms, thus keeping the body free of the harm caused by imbalances or destructive thoughts and emotions.

Quantum entanglement theory describes how particles engage in a continuous back and forth communication and effect each other even when separated by great distances, hinting at an explanation for distant healing. Einstein at first doubted that this theory could be true and called it *spooky action at a distance.* However, scientists continue to validate that it is true. Even thoughts can be picked up over great distances. Particles interact creating an unlimited amount of energy in the universe. It was once thought that outer space is a vacuum, an empty space devoid of anything. Now it is known that outer space is filled with energy as is the space all around us. This energy could potentially be harnessed as an energy source on earth, although harnessing it remains a challenge.

Although the connection between quantum physics and energy healing is still in its infancy, scientific terminology is a springboard for achieving some understanding of invisible phenomenon. While only some people can see subtle energy, in the 1970's Fritz-Albert Popp reported that all living things emit light as photons, stored in and emitted from DNA. Popp felt these photon emissions coordinated all cellular processes in the body.

The human energy field and the subtle energy generated in the healing process fall into the category of extremely low frequencies (ELF) requiring very sensitive equipment to detect it. In the 1980's Jon Zimmerman used a superconducting quantum interference device (SQUID) to detect frequencies emanating from an energy healer's hands as well as the energy frequencies active in different parts of the body.

I recall several classes during which Janet Mentgen used the term *electron transfer resonance* to describe how the process of Healing Touch healing might occur. The healer begins the process by working on the energy field outside the client's body, changing the vibrations of the energy. The vibration of the body's external field then resonates with and changes the frequencies of the skin. The effect progresses through the tissues of the body, re-balancing the energy of the skin, adipose, muscle, bone, and other tissues in succession. Although Janet was not a scientific researcher, her use of the term *electron transfer resonance* provides a working image of what might be occurring in the process of energy healing.

Research about the forces in the universe continues and is gradually bringing more understanding about how energy healing works. We can hope for more complete explanations of energy healing as we are even more awed by the wonders of creation.

Final Thoughts…With Gratitude

While energy healing demands a focus in the present moment, the work brings visions of what could be possible for humans in the future. We live in an amazing time when there is access to vast resources for self-development. Teachings once available only to holy ones or privileged individuals are now easily obtained by those ready to pursue deeper wisdom. Avatars, saints, mystics, and healers are living hidden in our midst. Yet, each person can increase their vibration to have a positive impact on helping others and transforming the world. Gaining the discipline in using that skill is moving the human race closer to a shift in values, perhaps away from materialism toward universal respect. Sensing that we are all connected as humans allows for true compassion. Political and economic solutions have not been successful in solving many global problems; perhaps energy healing can help transform power and control issues and lead more effectively to cooperation and peaceful resolution of conflicts. Let us hold these intentions and enjoy the miracles.

ADDENDUM A

How Healing Touch is different from a number of energy approaches:

- Includes the techniques of many healers
- Based in professional nursing practice, therefore uses assessments, planning, re-assessments, documentation
- Knowledge based: uses body of literature
- Uses research for evidence based practice
- Standardized curriculum
- Ethics and standards of practice
- Grounding
- Use of Intention
- Certification
- Mentorship/apprenticeship
- Emphasizes the importance of community
- Promotes personal and professional development of the practitioner
- Encourages self care for practitioner and client

ADDENDUM B

Safety and comfort when using a portable massage table

Although not everyone uses a massage table for energy treatments, the use of a table greatly helps the energy worker stay in physical alignment with minimal bending and strain. The following are guidelines for using a massage table safely and for maximum comfort of the client.

1) Be sure the surface of the table is level, with all table legs adjusted to the correct height for the practitioner and all cable supports aligned according to the design.
2) Tighten all screws and nuts on the table legs.
3) Clear area around the table to prevent tripping. Be sure there is enough room around the table to do the work you intend, e.g. working at the head or foot or either side.
4) Prepare the area before client arrives, setting in place sheet, pillowcase, bolsters, headrest and other props that will be used. Have water available for the client to drink after the session. Consider using a small table for documentation forms, water, etc.
5) Avoid leaning on or moving a portable table by yourself since it may weaken the legs. Have one person hold each end while moving. To move a table on your own, use furniture movers (tiny plastic discs) or turn it on its side and fold it up before moving it.
6) Have a step stool available for the client to step up to the table. Direct the client to sit on the table and then lay down. Being on the table on all fours is not safe.

7) Have pillows or bolsters available for under head and knees if client prefers them for comfort. A narrow pillow or rolled towel may be comfortable behind the neck. Some people are not comfortable lying face up or face down. It is worth taking the time to offer comfortable positioning to maximize relaxation and benefits of the treatment. If a client gets restless on the table, check in with them to see if they need repositioning. You may need to give them treatment on their side or sitting in a chair.

8) Some individuals are not comfortable using a headrest when lying face down. Try alternate positioning for lying face down. One example might be to have one arm resting on the table extended along the side of the head with a pillow under the shoulder and the other arm along the side of the body. The head is turned toward the upward arm in this position. Note: let the person choose what will work best for them. Let them know they can change positions as frequently as needed.

9) To relieve tension in muscles, stretch before and after giving treatments.

Use of other furniture

If not using a massage table, be sure whatever chair, bed, recliner, couch, or other surface used is safe and positioned as well as possible for comfort, with extra furniture out of the way. Keep the floor clear and safe from tripping hazards. If needed, use a chair to make the treatment easier for you. Try to keep your back straight, especially when holding positions for several minutes or longer.

REFERENCES

Preface

Ferguson, Marilyn. *The Aquarian Conspiracy: Personal and Social Transformation in the 1980s*. New York, NY: J. P. Tarcher Inc./Houghton Mifflin, 1980.

King, Godfré, R. *Unveiled Mysteries*. Schaumburg, Illinois: Saint Germain Foundation, 1934, reprinted 2001.

MacRitchie, James. *Chi Kung: Cultivating Personal Energy*. Rockport, MA: Element Books, Inc., 1993.

Roberts, Jane. *Seth Speaks: The Eternal Validity of the Soul*. San Rafael, CA by Amber-Allen Publishing, 1972, reprinted 1994

Saraswati, Satyananda. *Yoga Nidra*. Munger, Bihar, India: Yoga Publications Trust, 1976.

Shucman, Helen. *A Course in Miracles*. Farmingdale, NY: Foundation for Inner Peace. 1975.

Thie, John. *Touch for Health: The Complete Edition*. Camarillo, CA: De Vorss & Company, 2005.

Chapter 3

Brennan, Barbara A. *Hands of Light: A Guide to Healing Through the Human Energy Field.* New York, NY: Bantam Books, 1988.

Bruyere, Rosalyn. *Wheels of Light: Chakras, Auras, and the Healing Energy of the Body.* NY, New York: Fireside, 1994.

Eden, Donna. *Energy Medicine.* New York, NY: Jeremy P. Tarcher, 1998.

Myss, Caroline. *Anatomy of the Spirit: The Seven Stages of Power and Healing.* New York, NY: Random House, Inc., 1997.

Chapter 6

Bailey, Alice. *Esoteric Healing.* Seventeenth Reprinting in 2012. New York, NY: Lucis Publishing Company, 1953.

Chapter 7

Benjamin, Ben E. and Sohnen-More, Cherie. *The Ethics of Touch.* Tucson, AZ: SMA Inc, 2005.

Feinstein, David and Eden, Donna. *Ethics Handbook for Energy Healing Practitioners.* Fulton, CA: Energy Psychology Press, 2011.

Hover-Kramer, D. *Creating Right Relationships: A Practical Guide to Ethics in Energy Therapies.* Cave Junction, OR: Behavioral Health Consultants, 2005.

Taylor, Kylea. *The Ethics of Caring: Honoring the Web of Life in Our Professional Healing Relationships.* Santa Cruz, CA: Hanford Mead Publishers, 1995.

Chapter 9

Byrne, Rhonda. *The Secret.* New York: NY: Atria Books, 2006.

Chapter 11

Craig, Gary. *Six Days at the VA*. Emotional Freedom Technique Course on DVD part 1, video 3,1994. www.emofree.com.

Gendlin, Eugene *Focusing*. New York, NY: Bantam Books. 1982.

Herman, Judith. *Trauma and Recovery: The Aftermath of Violence — from Domestic Abuse to Political Terror*. New York, NY: BasicBooks, a Division of HaperCollins Publishers, 1992.

Levine, Peter. *Waking the Tiger: Healing Trauma*. Berkeley, CA: North Atlantic Books, 1997.

Levine, Peter. *In an Unspoken Voice: How the Body Releases Trauma and Restores Goodness*. Berkeley, CA: North Atlantic Books 2010.

Naparstek, Belleruth. *Invisivble Heroes: Survivors of Trauma and How They Heal*. New York, NY: Bantam Books, 2004.

Naparstek, Bellaruth. *Healing Trauma*. Audio CD. Akron, OH: Healthjourneys.com, 1999.

Porges, Stephen. "Beyond the Brain: Using Polyvagal Theory to Help Patients 'Reset' the Nervous System after Trauma. Webinar Session October 15, 2014 through the National Institute for the Clinical Application of Behavioral Medicine.

Scaer, Robert. *The Trauma Spectrum: Hidden Wounds and Human Resiliency*. New York, NY: WW Norton & Company, 2005.

Jain, S., McMahon, G., Hasen, P., Kozub, A., Porter, V., King, R., Guarneri, E. "Healing Touch with Guided Imagery for PTSD in Returning Active Duty Military: A Randomized Controlled Trial. *Military Medicine*, vol. 177, Sept, 2012.

Chapter 12

Benor, Daniel. "Distant Healing" *Subtle Energies and Energy Medicine*, 2000, 11(3), p. 249.

Vitale, Joe and Ihaleakala, Hew Len. *Zero Limits: The Secret Hawaiian System for Wealth, Health, Peace, and More.* Hoboken, NJ: John Wiley & Sons, Inc., 2007.

Chapter 14

Achterberg, Jeanne. *Imagery in Healing: Shamanism and Modern Medicine.* Boston, MA: Shambala Publications, 1985.

Benor, Daniel. *Spiritual Healing: A Scientific Validation of a Healing Revolution.* Southfield, MI: Vision Publications, 2001.

Bingen, Hildegarde. *Illuminations of Hildegard of Bingen.* Text by Hildegard of Bingen with commentary by Matthew Fox. Santa Fe, NM: Bear & Company,1985.

Childre, Doc and Rozman, Deborah. *Transforming Stress: The Heartmath Solution for Relieving Worry, Fatigue, and Tension.* Oakland, CA: New Harbinger Publications, Inc., 2005.

Dossey, Barbara, Keegan, Lynn, and Guzzetta, Cathie. *Holistic Nursing: A Handbook for Practice.* Third edition. Gaithersburg, MD: Aspen Publishers, Inc., 2000.

Goleman, Daniel. *Mind-Body Medicine: How to Use Your Mind for Better Health.* Yonkers, NY: Consumer Reports Books, 1993.

Gordon, Richard. *Quantum-Touch: The Power to Heal — Introduction to Quantum-Touch and Extraordinary New Ways to Run Life Force Energy with Quantum-Touch.* VHS tape recordings, Santa Cruz, CA: Quantum-Touch, 2002.

Guarneri, Mimi. *The Heart Speaks: A Cardiologist Reveals the Secret Language of Healing.* New York, NY: Touchstone, 2006.

Joy, Brugh. *Joy's Way: A Map for the Transformational Journey. An Introduction to the Potentials for Healing with Body Energies.* Los Angeles, CA: JP Tarcher, Inc., 1979.

Lipton, Bruce *The Biology of Belief: Unleashing the Power of Consciousness, Matter and Miracles.* New York, NY: Hay House, Inc. (2005

McTaggart, Lynne. *The Field: The Quest for the Secret Force of the Universe.* New York: NY: HarperCollins Publishers, 2002.

Meggs, William J. *The Inflammation Cure: Simple Steps for Reversing Heart Disease, Arthritis, Asthma, Diabetes, Alzheimer's Disease, Osteoporosis, and Other Diseases of Aging.* McGraw-Hill Education, 2005.

Simonton, O. Carl and Matthews-Simonton, Stephanie, and Creighton, James L. *Getting Well Again.* New York, NY: Bantam Books, 1978.

Szczepanski, Mary. *Strands.* Bloomington, IN: iUniverse, 2014

ADDITIONAL RESOURCES

For information about setting up classes in energy healing, Healing Touch, Emotional Freedom Technique (EFT) and related classes in your area, contact Mary Szczepanski at HealingTouchAlaska.com.

INDEX